John A. D'addario
2244 Esplanade
The Bronx, M.Y 10469
798 - 0560
AECOM mail box #255

The Biology of
Cancer

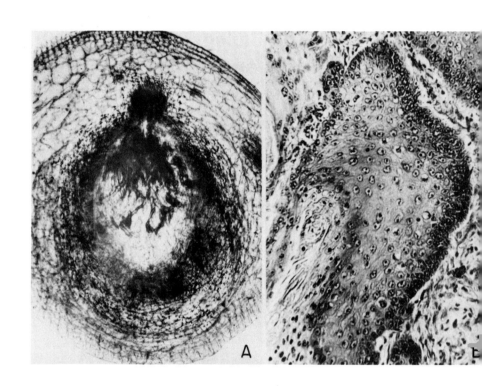

This figure, also reproduced on p. 119 with detailed caption, illustrates the partial self-
healing of tumors in the plant and animal fields.
In both instances the tumor cells may undergo a
form of terminal differentiation resulting spontaneously in a loss of the tumorous properties.
(Courtesy of Dr. Roy E. Albert)

The Biology of Cancer

Armin C. Braun
The Rockefeller University

1974
Addison-Wesley Publishing Company
Advanced Book Program
Reading, Massachusetts

London · Amsterdam · Don Mills, Ontario · Sydney · Tokyo

Library of Congress Cataloging in Publication Data

Braun, Armin C   1911-
   The biology of cancer.

   Includes bibliographical references and index.
   1. Cancer. 2. Cancer cells. I.   Title.
[DNLM: 1. Neoplasms.   QZ200 B827b]
RC263.B64   616.9'94'07   74-20895
ISBN 0-201-00764-9
ISBN 0-201-00765-7 pbk.

Reproduced by Addison-Wesley Publishing Company, Inc., Advanced Book Program, Reading, Massachusetts, from camera-ready copy prepared by the author.

Manufactured in the United States of America

CONTENTS

PREFACE

This book was written not for the specialist but rather for a beginner who has acquired a background in the basic biological sciences and who is interested in gaining insight into our present understanding of the cancer problem. The biology of cancer is examined here in the broadest terms and an attempt is made not only to identify the essential biological concepts that underlie the tumorous state but to critically evaluate as well the premises upon which prevailing thought in the field of experimental oncology is based.

Cancer research has quite understandably focused very heavily throughout the past century on proximate causes and cures, while relatively little attention has been paid until quite recently toward gaining an understanding of the basic cellular mechanisms that underlie the tumorous state. If an understanding of cancer is ultimately to be achieved, the experimental oncologist will have to explain why cancer cells divide persistently and in an unrestrained manner in their hosts and why such cells invade underlying normal tissues and metastasize to distant sites, while the growth of all normal cells is precisely regulated. These are dynamic problems that will ultimately find their explanation in terms of the specific substances and mechanisms that are involved in the regulation of growth. While an attempt was made in this general survey to cover, albeit briefly, most if not all aspects of cancer biology, emphasis has been placed here on those investigations that appear most likely to provide insight into an understanding of that problem. This was done not only to stress the purpose and significance of pertinent studies that bear on these matters but, more importantly perhaps, to provide a conceptual framework for possible future inves-

tigations in this challenging and most important
area of the scientific endeavor.

Armin C. Braun

The Biology of
Cancer

CHAPTER I

INTRODUCTION

INTRODUCTORY REMARKS

It has recently been estimated that of the
somewhat more than 200 million people now alive in
the United States, some 50 million will develop
cancer and, of these, 34 million will die of that
disease unless more adequate methods than are now
available can be found to cope with that disorder
(143). In addition to being a medical problem of
greatest urgency, cancer represents one of the
most fundamental and challenging areas for study
in the basic biological sciences and one in which
the knowledge and skills acquired in many different
disciplines will have to be applied if an understanding of that problem is to be achieved.

1

Cancer is a disease of cells and is, therefore, equally capable of expression in all higher
organisms. It is thus a problem of unusually
broad scope which offers a wide choice of experimental test organisms for study. Included among
these are certain higher plant species, frogs,
chickens, mice, hamsters, and numerous other mammalian systems, each of which has in its own way
and because of its own unique characteristics con-
tributed importantly to our present understanding
of the basic cellular mechanisms that underlie the
tumorous state.

DISTINGUISHING CHARACTERISTICS OF TUMOR CELLS. In
setting out to analyze a problem as complex as the
tumor problem it would appear necessary to first
clearly define the distinguishing characteristics
of the tumorous state and then to critically
evaluate the premises upon which prevailing thought
is based. What, then, are the distinguishing
characteristics of tumor cells in general and of
malignant cells in particular?

A tumor cell, whether benign or malignant,
is a persistently altered cell that reproduces

true to type and against the growth of which there
is no adequate control mechanism in a host. The
implication of that statement is that during the
transition from a normal cell to a tumor cell a
profound and heritable change occurs which allows
a tumor cell to determine its own activities
largely irrespective of the laws that govern so
precisely the growth of all normal cells in an
organism. This newly acquired property, which is
known as autonomy, is the most important single
characteristic of tumor cells since without it
there would be no tumors. A second characteristic
that is common to both benign and malignant tumors
is that of transplantability. When true tumor
cells are removed from a host or taken from cell
culture and implanted into an appropriate host of
the same species they develop again into tumorous
growths identical to those from which the tumor
cells were derived. Whether a tumor cell is transplantable depends, in part at least, on the degree
of autonomy that that cell has achieved. Two
clinically important characteristics that distinguish malignant from benign tumors are the ability
of the former to invade underlying tissues and to

detach small groups of cells from the tumorous mass which then move, or metastasize, through the blood vessels and lymph channels to distant sites where new tumors may arise. It is this capacity of malignant cells to become widely disseminated in a host that makes cancer such a dangerous and often incurable disease. It may be noted, however, that certain tumors of the endocrine glands (e.g., islet cell, adrenal and extraadrenal chromaffin tissue tumors) may be highly toxic or even lethal when only microscopic in size due to an excessive secretion of their specific hormones. Such tumors, although sometimes lethal, may show limited cell divisions and may not invade or metastasize during the early period of their development. These tumors are malignant in the sense that they may kill their hosts and yet they remain localized at the time that they secrete their lethal products. Benign tumors are by definition those that remain localized at the site of origin in their hosts. The capacities to grow autonomously, to invade and to metastasize are, however, dissociable characters (59). There are, for example, certain tumors that invade underlying normal tissues deeply but rarely

metastasize, while others become widely distributed
in their hosts despite a minimum of local invasion
while still others, although transplantable, do not
commonly invade or metastasize but, rather, con-
tinue to grow autonomously, reaching huge size and
ultimately cause death by simply overwhelming their
hosts. (See Fig. 1) These last-mentioned tumors
(e.g., keratomas) occasionally give rise to cells
that invade and metastasize and thus become malignant in the clinical sense. The capacities to invade and metastasize may thus be acquired, sometimes relatively late, and may therefore be dis-
missed in a search for the earliest event responsible for the alteration of a normal cell to a
tumor cell which, as has been indicated, is the
acquisition by a tumor cell of a capacity for autonomous growth. Autonomy is not, however, a fixed
and unvarying character but has many gradations
ranging from very slowly to very rapidly growing
tumor cell types. It should be noted, however,
that even some of the most rapidly growing tumor
cells do not grow at a faster rate than do certain
normal cell types. When, for example, three-fourths
of a normal liver is removed surgically, the remain-

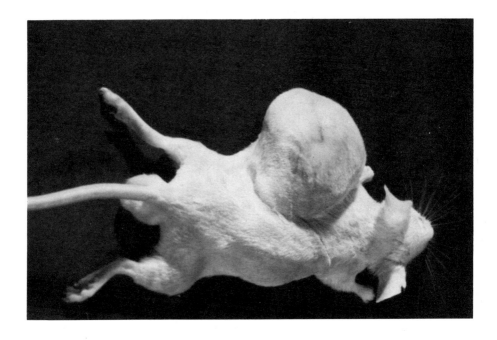

Fig. 1. A transplantable tumor (keratoma) of the
type that does not invade neighboring tissues and
does not metastasize but overwhelms and ultimately
kills its host as a result of continued growth.
This type of tumor occasionally gives rise to cells
that invade and metastasize and thus becomes malignant in the clinical sense. The capacities to
invade and metastasize may thus be acquired, sometimes relatively late, and may therefore be dis-
missed in a search for the earliest event responsible for the conversion of a normal cell to a
tumor cell. (Courtesy of Dr. James S. Henderson)

ing liver cells will regenerate the complete organ
in about two weeks time. Tumors of the liver sel-
dom achieve comparable growth rates. It is thus
not rate of growth that is important to the tumor
problem, but, rather, the development of a capacity
for unrestrained or autonomous growth.

The significant concept that tumorigenesis
may in certain instances occur as a multistep process, progressing by a series of continuous (gradual)
or discontinuous (abrupt) changes from the benign
to the malignant state, is now well established and
Foulds (47) has proposed six general principles
underlying this phenomenon which has come to be
known as tumor progression. In multistage tumor
development a chemical carcinogen may convert normal cells into tumor cells which do not as yet proliferate into a tumorous growth. Such tumor cells
require another type of chemical (e.g., croton oil),
which is called a promoter or cocarcinogen, to
stimulate the incipient tumor cells to develop into
a neoplastic growth. Each stage in the multistage
process may be facilitated by specific chemicals
that may not be active as promoters at other stages.
In other instances the transformation of a normal

cell into a fully autonomous, rapidly growing tumor
cell appears to occur as a single step.

Another distinguishing characteristic of
tumor cells is their lack of perfect form and function. This loss of certain cellular characters is
known as anaplasia and represents a dedifferentiation of the tumor cells. Dedifferentiation is sometimes erroneously looked upon as representing a
reversion of the tumorous state to the embryonic
state. While it is true that tumor cells may acquire, as a result of their transformation, a capacity to produce certain proteins (fetal antigens)
which are characteristic of embryonic cells but are
not commonly found in the somatic cells from which
the tumors were derived, they do not resemble embryonic cells as far as their growth characteristics
are concerned. Normal embryonic cells, even in
their most undifferentiated form, respond beautifully to the control mechanisms provided by the
organism and by one another while dedifferentiated
cancer cells respond poorly to those controls. The
generality of tumor cells are not, however, completely anarchic and the growths that they form are
not completely chaotic, indicating that such cells

do respond in part, at least, to the influences that regulate the growth of normal cells within an organism. Finally it should be pointed out that how a tumor develops in a host may be determined by the environment in which that tumor is growing. This is particularly well illustrated in the so-called conditional or hormone-dependent tumors of animals and plants. Conditional prostate or breast tumors of mammals, which may be highly malignant, grow only so long as the appropriate hormonal stimulus is present. When the specific stimulus is withdrawn growth of the tumors stops and they regress, but when the stimulus is restored tumors will reoccur in the same place and with the same characteristics that they originally showed. Many conditional tumors undergo progression to a hormone-independent state and then become true tumors.

THE CAUSES OF CANCER. One of the most puzzling aspects of the tumor problem is concerned with the multiplicity of diverse physical, chemical, and biological agencies that are capable of converting normal cells into tumor cells. An almost endless catalogue of agents, which include among others such physical oncogens as ultraviolet light, X-rays, radium, plutonium, strontium 89, and iodine 131, has been shown to be effective in initiating cancers (99). It has also been found that plastics of various types when implanted into tissues as films evoke the formation of sarcomas (connective tissue tumors) in rats (107). The fact that stainless steel films are also effective suggests that some physical condition rather than a chemical reaction is responsible for the sarcomatous change in these instances.

Among the inorganic substances shown to be effective oncogens are arsenic, asbestos, chromate-, cobalt-, and nickel-containing compounds. Numerous organic substances which range from structurally relatively simple compounds such as urethane (ethyl carbamate) to the cross-linking agents (e.g., ethylene amine), the alkylating oncogens (e.g., NN-di(2-chloroethyl)methyl amine) to the structurally complex heterocyclic hydrocarbons (e.g., methylcholanthrene), many of which contain five fused rings in their molecule, have all been found to be effective oncogens. Substances present in chimney soot, gas works tars, tobacco, and certain coal tar dye intermediates as β-naphthylamine, diphenylamine, and benzidine have also been found to be effective oncogens, as are the aflatoxins which are a product of metabolism of the fungus species <u>Aspergillus flavus</u>. Such naturally occurring body substances as the estrogens have, moreover, been shown to be effective in eliciting a variety of tumors when administered to experimental animals.

Of the approximately 1,000 different chemical substances that have now been shown to be oncogenic, a considerable number are found in the biosphere. It has been estimated that 70% or more of all tumors that arise in man are caused by such environmental oncogens. It is imperative, therefore, that they be identified and eliminated from the environment in so far as that is possible in modern industrial societies. Prevention is unquestionably the most effective method of dealing with cancer at the present time.

There are numerous instances in which peculiar customs practiced by members of certain societies have led directly to a high incidence of cancer and which, once identified as being etiologically in-volved, could easily be eliminated by simply discon-

tinuing that practice (63). There were and perhaps
still are, for example, the betel nut chewers in
Travancore, on the southwest coast of India, who
mixed betel nuts with a cheap tobacco and lime from
crushed sea shells. It has been estimated that 75%
of the oral cancers diagnosed in Travancore were
attributable to the persistent chewing of such a
quid. This situation was aggravated further by the
finding that the diets of those individuals who
developed cancers were seriously deficient in vitamin A, - a vitamin that seems to be importantly
involved in establishing resistance to certain other
cancers. In Kashmir, on the other hand, it was a
common practice among the natives to bind small
charcoal-burning earthen ovens around their waists
during the cold periods of the year in order to warm
themselves. Cancers, which are known as Kanghri
ɔurn cancers, commonly developed on the abdominal
ʋall at the points of irritation produced by the
ιot earthen oven. Another curious custom, practiced
y certain individuals in south Asia, and known
ocally as chutta, is one that involves the smoking
f cigars with the lighted end in their mouths.
ιis practice resulted in a very high incidence of

oral cancers. A strong positive correlation has
also been found to exist between the clay pipe
smokers in Ireland and cancer of the lip. Oral
cancers are, moreover, significantly more prevalent
among habitual snuff users than they are in the
general population. The relationship that exists
between heavy cigarette smokers and lung cancer now
appears well established. Here one finds, however,
that the incidence of lung cancer is far higher
among cigarette smokers working in the asbestos industry than among cigarette smokers in the general
population. This disease also appears to be more
prevalent among cigarette smokers living in an urban
industrial environment than in a rural environment,
suggesting again that a combination of factors may
be etiologically involved here. There are, moreover,
sufficiently large differences in the cancer incidence between urban and rural non-smokers to indicate that carcinogens present in the atmosphere and
resulting from the combustion of fuels play a significant role in the development of lung and perhaps
other cancers as well.

It has long been recognized that prolonged
exposure to strong sunlight and particularly the

ultraviolet region of the spectrum leads to the development of certain types of skin cancer. This relationship was first clearly recognized in the last century when attention was called to the high incidence of skin cancer among sailors following prolonged exposure to strong sunlight.

The first occupational cancer was, however, recognized almost 200 years ago when Percival Pott, in England, reported that the then commonly used practice of lowering very small boys down chimneys to clean them resulted in a high incidence of scrotal cancer due presumably to prolonged exposure to the irritating effects of the soot (111). With the development of the coal tar industry in the latter part of the last century an abundance of clinical evidence became available implicating certain by-products of that industry as causative agents in the genesis of cancers. Rehn (113), among others, reported a high incidence of cancer of the bladder among workers in the aniline dye industry. Since that time numerous studies have implicated specific substances characteristically associated with specific occupations as being etiologically involved in the causation of cancer (54, 69). The development

of lung cancers, for example, was found much more
commonly among workers who inhaled dust from chro-
mate ores or those who worked in the asbestos industry than in the general population, while workers
in nickel refining plants developed cancers of the
nasal sinuses. Another tragic example, that could
have been easily avoided had the consequences been
known, is found in the case of the women who painted
luminous dials on watches by dipping their brushes
into a dilute radium-containing solution and then
pointing those brushes in their mouths. Many developed cancer of the bone as a result of the prolonged use of this practice. As this is being
written vinyl chloride, a gaseous chemical used in
the plastics industry, has been linked to the development of a rather rare type of tumor (angiosarcoma)
of the liver in a number of workers in different
plastic manufacturing plants. These are but some
of the many examples of this type which, once recognized, either have been or could easily be avoided
with the use of the proper protective measures. The
importance of establishing a relationship between
the occurrence of certain cancers and exposure to
specific environmental factors is obvious. By

application of such knowledge many cancers now arising in man can doubtless be prevented.

Although certain of the chemical carcinogens have been shown to be cancer-producing without structural modification, many others require structural changes in their molecules before their ultimate active forms are realized. They must be activated enzymatically within a target cell so that they contain electron-deficient atoms (strong electrophiles) in their molecules which then react chemically with the electron-rich atoms (strong nucleophiles) found in the nucleic acids and proteins of a cell (98). Two examples of the enzymatic reactions that are believed to be required for the conversion of a carcinogen to its ultimate active form are shown in Fig. 2. Whether cells of a particular tissue become converted into tumor cells would appear to depend, in part at least, on whether the appropriate enzymes needed to convert a carcinogen to its ultimate active form are present in or can be induced in those cells. It has been found in preliminary studies, for example, that approximately 9% of the white population in the United States has a capacity for the induction in

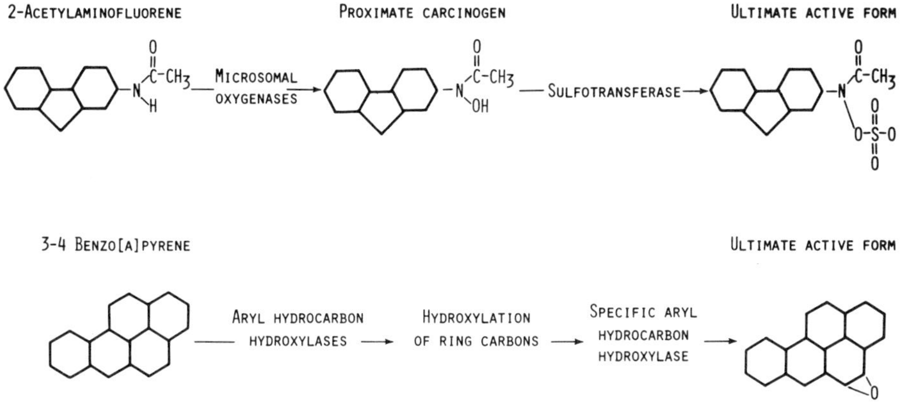

2-ACETYLAMINOFLUORENE   PROXIMATE CARCINOGEN   ULTIMATE ACTIVE FORM

3-4 BENZO[A]PYRENE   ULTIMATE ACTIVE FORM

Fig. 2. Two examples of the enzymatic reactions
that are believed to be required to convert a
carcinogen into its ultimate active form.

lymphocytes of high concentrations of aryl hydro-

carbon hydroxylases, the enzymes that convert poly-

cyclic hydrocarbons to their ultimate active forms.

Moderate concentrations of these enzymes were found

to be inducible in about half of the population,

while low induction rates were found in the others

(74, 75, 93). It was reported further that the in-

cidence of lung cancer was about 36% higher in ciga-

rette smokers with high enzyme inducibility, about

16% higher in those with moderate inducibility than

in those individuals whose cells showed low enzyme

inducibility. In these studies the induction of
aryl hydrocarbon hydroxylases was measured in lymphocytes rather than in cells of the lung and the
assumption was made that the two types of cells
respond similarly. If, nevertheless, further more
extensive surveys show a similar relationship to
exist it may be possible for the first time to determine in advance those individuals who are most
likely to develop lung cancer from smoking ciga-
rettes or from other causes.

In addition to the numerous physical and
chemical agents shown to be tumor-producing, biological entities of the most diverse type including,
among others, bacteria, animal parasites of several
kinds, as well as viruses, have been found to elicit
tumors in higher organisms. Of these the viruses
are by far the most important etiologically and
approximately 150 different viruses have now been
shown to induce tumors in animals and plants. The
oncogenic viruses, like the generality of viruses,
may contain either DNA or RNA as their nucleic acid
component. Certain of the oncogenic viruses (SV40,
polyoma) contain only enough genetic information to
code for between four and eight proteins, depending

on their size, while others (Rous sarcoma virus)
possess enough information to code for two dozen or
so proteins. Some of these oncogenic viruses have
a very limited host range (Shope papilloma virus)
and induce only one type of tumor in a single animal
species, while others (polyoma virus) have a much
wider host range and elicit the formation of many
different and distinct kinds of tumors in a given
host. Some oncogenic viruses (mouse mammary tumor
virus, Shope papilloma virus) initiate the formation
of only benign tumors many of which may and commonly
do give rise to malignant derivatives when growing
in appropriate hosts. The mouse mammary tumor
virus, for example, has been found to be only one
of several factors involved in a very complex etiology. In addition to the virus, both hormonal influences and an inherited breast cancer susceptibility
are important factors that determine whether a
malignant tumor will develop. Other oncogenic
viruses (Rous sarcoma virus) transform cells directly into rapidly growing, fully autonomous tumor cell
types. It is clear therefore that the oncogenic
viruses represent a heterogeneous group of disease-
producing entities the common denominator of which

is an ability to elicit the formation of tumors in
appropriate host species.

The central problems in cells transformed by
the oncogenic viruses are (1) to define the exact
form of the association that develops between a
virus and a target cell, and (2) to characterize
the metabolic changes that occur in a cell following
transformation and that results in a capacity by a
tumor cell for autonomous growth. Both of these
questions will be considered in some detail later
in this discussion.

In addition to the physical, chemical, and
biological carcinogens, it has been found that
cancer cells may arise as a result of growing normal cells for prolonged periods in culture under
conditions in which no known carcinogen has to be
added to a culture medium in order to achieve the
neoplastic transformation (37, 50).

We are thus confronted with a most perplexing
situation. The transformation of a normal cell
to a cancer cell may occur in culture without the
influence of any recognizable carcinogen, it may
be accomplished by physical agents, by very simple
inorganic or organic compounds, by more complex

organic molecules, and by very complex biological
agents such as the viruses. Is there, then, some
common denominator that can account for these un-
usual observations? The answer is probably yes and
if that is true it must be looked for in the nature
of the heritable cellular change which, in turn, is
reflected in that area of metabolism that is concerned with the regulation of cell growth and division.

HEREDITARY FACTORS. In addition to the multiplicity
of proximate causes shown to be effective in eliciting tumors, the genetic constitution of a host
appears to be of central importance in determining
whether or not a tumor will be initiated. This is
evidenced most clearly in the high- and low-incidence
lines of inbred strains of mice where in the high-
incidence lines virtually every member will die of
cancer at a predestined time, and even the very site
of the origin of the new growth is commonly prede-
termined. The conclusion to be drawn from the very
extensive genetic studies on mice carried on during
the past half century is that all types of mouse
cancer thus far investigated have some genetic

basis (88). Although man can obviously not be subjected to experimental breeding there is every reason to believe that there is a strong heritable factor determining cancer-proneness in man as well as
in the mouse. This is perhaps most clearly shown
in studies of identical twins. Identical twins are
two individuals endowed with identical heredity and
this important component is therefore a constant
factor within any pair of twins. In one study twen-
ty reports of tumors of various types occurring in
identical twins were collected (95). In every case
reported the tumor was present in each twin of a
pair and it was, moreover, of the same type, occurring in the same tissue or organ. Since the twins
were not usually living together and were often many
miles apart and thus not subjected to the same environmental conditions, these findings appear to be
more than coincidence. It should be emphasized,
however, that members of an identical twin pair do
not always both develop tumors, and many instances
have been reported in which one twin develops a
particular type of tumor whereas the other does not.
Certain types of tumors show no significant difference in concordance between identical and fraternal

twins, suggesting that genetic predisposition to
them is negligible.

An analysis of human pedigrees has demonstrated
that a proneness for the development of certain
types of tumors is determined genetically, sometimes
by single alleles. Xeroderma pigmentosum, for
example, has been found to result from a recessive
and partially sex-linked gene. The skin of persons
homozygous for this recessive gene invariably develops malignant tumors but only if exposed to strong
sunlight or other forms of radiation. What is obviously transmitted in this instance is not the cancer
but the gene which then predisposes the skin exposed
to sunlight to the development of cancer.

Finally, crosses between related species of
animals or plants sometimes result in hybrids that
develop tumors spontaneously and in large numbers.
The most thoroughly studied examples of this type
are the melanomas that develop regularly in back
crosses of the F_1 hybrids of platyfish X swordtail
in fish (57) and the spontaneous tumors that arise
regularly in certain interspecific hybrids in plants
of the genus Nicotiana (128) (See Fig. 8). An
interesting example is also found when the wild

mouse and an inbred strain of the domestic mouse
are crossed. Here the incidence of tumors in the
hybrid is tenfold higher than is the sum of the
parental incidence (87).

Tumors that develop as a result of hybridization may be considered to support the so-called
chromosomal imbalance theory of cancer in which
genetic imbalance is expressed in developmental
imbalance.

Before leaving this section on cancer causation it should be noted that the so-called oncogenic
agents such as the carcinogenic chemicals as well
as X-rays and other forms of radiation are concerned
only with the inception of tumors and play no role
in the continued abnormal or autonomous proliferation of the tumor cells once the cellular transformation has been accomplished. A part or all of the
genetic information introduced in a cell by the
oncogenic viruses appears, on the other hand, to be
required for both the inception and maintenance of
the tumorous state in virally transformed cells.
This knowledge, in itself, tells us nothing about
the cellular changes which are the immediate cause
of malignant behavior. It would appear necessary

therefore to determine the nature of the heritable
cellular changes at a physiological and biochemical
level if an understanding of the basic cellular
mechanisms that underlie the tumorous state is to
be achieved.

CHAPTER II

THE DEVELOPMENT OF AUTONOMY

AUTONOMY IN PLANT AND ANIMAL CELLS

While a great deal of effort has quite understandably been devoted in the past to a study of
the causes of cancer and to its cure, very little
definitive work has been reported until quite
recently concerning the basic cellular mechanisms
that underlie the tumorous state. The cancer
problem, regardless of the initiating cause, is
fundamentally a dynamic problem of abnormal and
autonomous cell growth and division. The transformation of a normal cell into a tumor cell must
involve a profound and persistent switch in the
pattern of synthesis going from the precisely regulated metabolism, which is concerned with differen-

26

tiated function and which is characteristic of a
normal resting cell, to one involving the continued
synthesis of the nucleic acids, the mitotic and
enzymatic proteins as well as other substances that
are concerned rather specifically with cell growth
and division (133). A rapidly growing, fully autonomous tumor cell may, in fact, be described as
a highly efficient proliferating system the energy
of which is directed largely toward a synthesis of
substances required for cell growth and division.
Because of the pronounced deterioration of form and
function (anaplasia) that such cancer cells show it
is often difficult for a pathologist to determine
the precise cell type from which the tumor arose.
This does not, of course, necessarily mean that the
factors that determine the pattern of metabolism
that is concerned with differentiated function are
lost by such cells; they may be present but simply
not be expressed. Such extreme dedifferentiation
is not the general rule, however, and most tumor
cells retain a sufficient capacity for differentiation and function that they are readily identifiable
as to the cell type of their origin and yet possess
a capacity for autonomous growth. At the other

extreme in this spectrum of examples is found the fastidious metabolism that is concerned with differentiated function and that is characteristic of a normal resting cell. It thus appears that two patterns of metabolism, the primitive of the tumor, which is involved with persistent cell growth and division, and the fastidious of the normal, which is concerned with differentiated function, compete with one another for ascendancy in a cell and the degree to which a cell is transformed would appear to determine the extent to which either pattern is expressed. This, then, brings us to the very fundamental question as to how these metabolic patterns are established and maintained in a cell and, thus, how a tumor cell acquires a capacity for autonomous growth. This is clearly a problem of growth, and growth in all higher organisms results either from an enlargement of cells or from the combined processes of cell enlargement and cell division.

REGULATION OF THE NORMAL CELL CYCLE. In order to understand how these fundamental growth processes are regulated in a cell we must turn our attention next to the normal cell cycle (See Fig. 3). In any

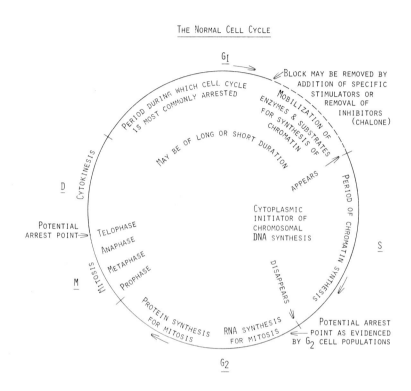

Fig. 3. Diagram of the normal cell cycle showing different phases of the cycle as well as potential arrest points.

proliferating population of cells the individual members commonly go through a cell cycle that consists of the now familiar phases that are designated as G_1, S, G_2, M, and D. The G_1 phase denotes that portion of interphase prior to the onset of chromosomal DNA replication. It is during that period

that there is a synthesis and mobilization of sub-
strates and enzymes required for nuclear DNA synthesis.   The G_1 phase is followed by a period of
chromosomal DNA and protein synthesis which is known
as the S phase of the cell cycle.   The G_2 phase
applies to that period between the end of chromosomal DNA synthesis and the onset of mitosis or nuclear division.   The mitotic process itself constitutes
the M phase of the cell cycle and it is during that
period that a precise distribution of the genetic
material in a dividing cell occurs.   Typically, although by no means universally, the end result of
mitosis is the production of two daughter cells by
a process known as cytokinesis.   This represents the
D phase of the cell cycle.   Following cell division,
the daughter cells again enter interphase where the
cell cycle may be arrested until appropriate stimuli
necessary to repeat the cycle are present.   The capacity of cells to regulate the sequence of events
that culminate in the division of one cell into two
is apparent.   It has indeed been suggested that a
cell that does not divide is a cell that is blocked
at some point in the cell cycle (94).   The implication of that statement, as far·as the present dis-

cussion is concerned, is that in any persistently
dividing population of cells such as those found in
tumors, all of the naturally occurring blocks are
removed, thus enabling such cells to divide continuously in an otherwise suitable environment. These
blocks include the G_1 phase block at which point the
normal cell cycle is most commonly arrested, the S
phase block which is determined in part by the absence of a cytoplasmic initiator of chromosomal DNA
synthesis, the G_2 block from which cells enter mitosis directly without again replicating their nuclear
DNA, and, finally, the block that occurs between
mitosis and cytokinesis. This is evidenced most
clearly by the rather common occurrence in both
animal and plant fields of the presence of binu-
cleate and multinucleate cells in which mitosis has
occurred without corresponding cell division. All
of the major blocks in the cell cycle appear to depend on the absence of some essential substance, or
at least they can be overcome by the addition of
specific substances. Yet, naturally occurring
tissue-specific substances inhibitory to cell division are synthesized by and have been isolated from
granulocytes, liver and kidney tissue, from mouse

ear epidermal cells, as well as a number of other
different and distinct cell types (67). These inhibitory substances, which are collectively known
as chalones, differ significantly from one another.
The liver chalone is a polypeptide of low molecular
weight (146) while the epidermal chalone is a basic
glycoprotein having a molecular weight of about
35,000 (66). The epidermal chalone is effective in
blocking the cell cycle only in the presence of
adrenalin (20). The evidence presented thus far
does not preclude the possibility that specific
stimulators of chromosomal DNA replication, mitosis,
and cytokinesis are synthesized by cells following
removal of the chalones. An antichalone has, in
fact, been isolated and has been shown to stimulate
division of granulocytes and to play an important
role in the control of their production (118). This
substance acts in the cell cycle prior to nuclear
DNA synthesis. It thus appears that the concepts
of specific stimuli versus specific inhibitors are
not necessarily mutually exclusive.

DEVELOPMENT OF AUTONOMY IN PLANT CELLS. How, then,
are these blocks that regulate events leading to

cell division in the normal cell cycle persistently
removed in tumor cells, thus enabling such cells to
grow and divide continuously in their hosts?   In
order to answer that question we might profitably
turn our attention to plant tumor systems for far
more is known in those systems than in animals.
Plant tumors are caused by the same general physical, chemical, and biological classes of agents
that cause tumors in animals (15).   Although, as
might be expected, there are some differences in
detail, tumors found in members of both kingdoms
have nevertheless much in common, and basic concepts developed with the use of the relatively
simple plant tumor systems could well find application and lead to an understanding of the tumor
problem generally.

Insight into the nature of autonomous growth
in plant tumor systems followed an understanding
of the nature of the substances that regulate normal cell growth and division.   Growth in all higher
animals and plants results either from an enlargement of cells or from the combined processes of
cell enlargement and cell division.   These fundamental growth processes are controlled in higher plant

species by the quantitative interaction of two
growth-regulating substances, the auxins, which are
concerned with cell enlargement and chromosomal DNA
replication, and the cell-division-promoting factors,
which act synergistically with the auxins to promote growth accompanied by cell division (17, 72)
(See Fig. 4). What appears to be an entirely analogous situation has recently been described in animals (125). In that study an as yet uncharacterized
dialyzable component has been implicated in chromosomal DNA synthesis, while a heat-labile, nondia-
lyzable substance has been found to act synergistically with the dialyzable component to promote mitosis and cytokinesis in the BHK21 line of hamster
cells grown in a serum-free medium. The nondia-
lyzable component, like the cell-division-promoting
factor in plants, is ineffective in encouraging
either DNA synthesis or in promoting cytokinesis in
the absence of the dialyzable factor.

It has been found that regardless of the initiating cause all true plant tumor cells thus far
studied are far less fastidious in their growth
requirements than are comparable normal cell types.
The plant tumor cells grow profusely and indefi-

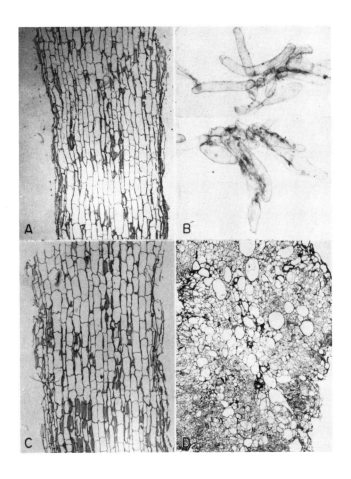

Fig. 4. The regulation of the processes of cell
enlargement and cell division in excised plant
parenchyma cells with the use of specific substances. Histological sections of: A, Untreated
control. B, Treated with an auxin (indole-3-acetic
acid) at a concentration of 1 mg/liter of medium.
Note cells have enlarged greatly without dividing.
C, Treated with a cell-division-promoting factor
(6-furfurylaminopurine) at a concentration of 0.5
mg/liter of medium. This compound does not promote
either cell enlargement or cell division in the
absence of auxin. D, Treated with both an auxin
(1 mg/liter) and the cell-division factor (0.5
mg/liter). Note growth accompanied by cell division
results from the synergistic effect of these two
growth-regulating substances.

nitely on a simple, chemically defined culture
medium composed only of mineral salts, sucrose and
three vitamins that does not support the continued
growth of normal cells. These studies show, further, that during the transition from a normal cell
to a tumor cell a series of quite distinct but well
defined biosynthetic systems, which represent the
entire area of metabolism concerned with cell growth
and division, become progressively and persistently
activated and the degree of activation of those systems within a tumor cell determines the rate at
which that cell type grows (13) (See Fig. 5). The
biosynthetic systems shown to be persistently activated may be divided operationally into two groups.
In the first group are the auxin and the cell-
division-promoting factor which establish the pattern of metabolism concerned with cell growth and
division and, because these two substances are synthesized persistently by the tumor cells, maintain
that pattern of synthesis in those cells. It is
those two substances that remove all of the blocks
that normally regulate the cell cycle in plants.

The second group of biosynthetic systems shown
to be persistently activated in plant tumor cells

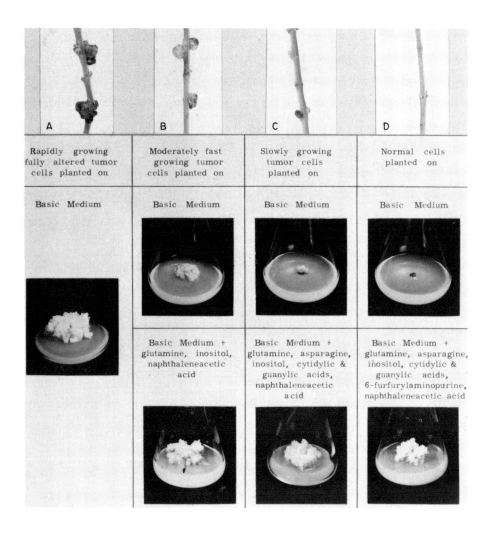

Fig. 5. The development of autonomy in the crown gall disease of Vinca rosea. Upper row: The transformation process was allowed to proceed for A, 72 hr; B, 60 hr; C, 34 hr; and D, control, after which times transformation was stopped. Middle row: Sterile tumor tissues isolated from tumors above and planted on a basic culture medium. Lower row: Pictures and legends show mineral nutrient requirements needed to achieve growth rates comparable to the fully autonomous tumor cells grown on the basic culture medium and shown at the left of the picture.

includes, among others, those responsible for the
production of such commonly found metabolites as
glutamine and asparagine, the purines and pyrimi-
dines, as well as myoinositol. Such metabolites
are required for the synthesis of the mitotic and
enzymatic proteins, the nucleic acids and, in the
case of myoinositol, the membrane systems of a cell.
These substances are needed to permit the pattern
of synthesis established in a cell by auxin and the
cell-division-promoting factor to be expressed.
Thus, plant tumor cells of several different kinds
develop a capacity for autonomous growth because
they have acquired, as a result of their transformation, a capacity to synthesize persistently the
two growth-regulating substances as well as the
essential metabolites that their normal counterparts
require for cell growth and division but cannot
themselves make.

In the crown gall disease of plants such a
persistent activation of biosynthetic systems
appears to be extensive and the tumor cells may
synthesize, in addition to the substances required
rather specifically for cell growth and division,
other substances that their normal counterparts

either do not produce or synthesize in only very
minute amounts. Interesting examples of this are
found in the three amino acid analogues, lysopine
(N^2-(D-1-carboxyethyl)-L-lysine), octopine (N^2-(D-
1-carboxyethyl)-L-arginine), and nopaline (N^2-(1,3-
dicarboxypropyl)-L-arginine), which are produced
in large amounts by the tumor tissues. These compounds were at first reported not to be synthesized
by normal cells, but a recent study using detection
methods far more sensitive than those originally
applied reported that very small amounts of these
substances are also synthesized by certain normal
plant cells (73).

Of particular interest is the finding that
octopine is synthesized in large amounts by certain
plant tumor tissues. This compound, which was
first isolated from octopus muscle and was reported
to be present only in octopus and related forms,
has now been found to be produced by plants. The
potentialities for the synthesis of that amino acid
were clearly carried through evolutionary development in the genome of many plant species but only
following the cellular transformation were those
potentialities fully expressed, leading to a sig-

nificant synthesis of that amino acid analogue by the transformed cells.

That a persistent activation of normally repressed biosynthetic systems may result in animal cells following their conversion to tumor cells is now widely recognized. It has been found, for example, that liver tumor cells contain an antigen which is identical to one present in embryonic tissue but is not found in normal adult liver (1). Similar results were obtained with a human gastrointestinal tumor (52, 53). The results of these studies indicate that genetic information that was expressed in the embryo was subsequently repressed following cellular differentiation and was again expressed in the liver and gastrointestinal tumors. Numerous other interesting examples are reviewed (49, 86) and these include the production of an ACTH-like substance by a primary carcinoma of the lung (92) and gonadotropin by a bronchogenic carcinoma (39). It is clear, therefore, that as the result of transformation the tumor cells may acquire biosynthetic capacities that are not expressed in their normal counterparts, suggesting that an extensive and persistent derepression of the cellular genome may occur during transformation.

DEVELOPMENT OF AUTONOMY IN ANIMAL CELLS. Can the
concepts that have been developed to explain autonomous growth of plant tumor cells be made to serve
as a model for animal cells as well? While differences in particulars will doubtless be found to
exist, there appears little in the animal litera-
ture that argues strongly against mechanisms involving the persistent activation of normally repressed
biosynthetic systems as the underlying basis of the
tumorous state in animal tumor systems. In order
to gain insight into this question it will be necessary to learn how the several blocks that regulate
the normal cell cycle are persistently removed during the conversion of a normal cell into an animal
tumor cell and thus to permit the tumor cell to grow
and divide continuously in an unrestrained manner.
The persistent removal of those blocks could be
accounted for if it could be shown that animal tumor
cells, but not comparable normal resting cells,
synthesize persistently, as indicated above, a small
molecular weight substance that is concerned with
chromosomal DNA replication and that acts synergis-

tically with a large molecular weight substance to promote cell growth and division in BHK21 cells in a serum-free culture medium. That the continued production of those substances by a tumor cell would not itself be sufficient to account for the continued abnormal proliferation of such cells is evidenced by the fact that the generality of animal tumor cells require either serum or plasma to be present in a culture medium for their continued growth. It should be noted, however, that tumor cells may require significantly lesser amounts of the serum factor(s) than do comparable normal cell types for optimal growth in culture (34, 35, 65, 122, 136, 140). Certain of these factors have now been characterized chemically (58). Thus, as in the case of auxin and the cell division factor in plants, the two substances found to regulate cell growth and division in BHK21 cells may simply establish the pattern of metabolism concerned with cell growth and division, while one or more substances present in serum or plasma may be required to permit that pattern of synthesis to be expressed.

That certain animal tumors (the desmoplasias) may actively synthesize powerful growth-promoting

substances is suggested by the fact that the normal
cells of the stroma adjacent to such tumors are
stimulated to very active division by the growing
tumor cells. This is evidenced further by the
recent finding of a so-called "overgrowth stimulating factor" which is found in a culture medium
in which Rous sarcoma virus-transformed cells are
growing (116). This interesting factor can cause
normal cells in culture to mimic the appearance
and growth habit of tumor cells. The treated cells
revert to the normal phenotype when the "overgrowth
stimulating factor" is absent from the medium. This
factor appears to be a proteolytic enzyme(s) and
its effects on growth can be reproduced with trypsin
or with pronase. Many tumors show high concentrations of such a proteolytic enzyme(s) at or near
their most actively growing cells. As well as being a growth-promoting factor, this substance may
contribute to or be responsible for the invasive-
ness of cancer cells. Recent studies have suggested
that two proteins, one secreted by the transformed cells (a protease) and the other present in
serum (plasminogen), interact to give rise to the
biologically active substance which has been given

the trivial name fibrinolysin (108, 144). It was

found, further, that tumor-bearing chickens, but

not normal chickens, contain an inhibitor that pre-

vents the action of the proteolytic enzyme(s). This

suggests that the inihibitor is formed in a host in

response to a tumor and that such an inhibitor may

play a part in the frequently observed regressions

of chicken sarcomas. The importance of the prote-

olytic enzyme(s) in the growth and development of

cancer cells of several types is evidenced by the

fact that the growth of those cells can be selec-

tively inhibited by a variety of known proteolytic

enzyme inhibitors (123).

The proteolytic enzyme(s) most probably

affects the surface properties of the normal cells

and thus alters the response of those cells to

exogenous regulatory substances which, in turn,

stimulate normal cells to active proliferation.

How, then, do such exogenous environmental factors

regulate the growth of normal cells and how may an

animal tumor cell acquire a capacity for autonomous

growth?

It is clear that success in characterizing

the nature of autonomy in plant tumor systems

depended largely on the development of a selective culture medium that permitted the profuse growth of tumor cells but not of comparable normal cell types. This same strategy has recently been applied to an animal tumor system in an attempt to gain insight into the basic cellular mechanisms that underlie autonomy in that system (3). An attempt was made in that study to reproduce as closely as possible in cell culture the conditions as they are known to exist in an animal host. A number of criteria that were believed to be essential if success was to be achieved were applied to this system. Those criteria were the following: (1) Blood plasma was used in place of serum. Although serum is almost universally used in culture media and is known to contain substances that promote cell division, it is not serum but plasma that normally nourishes cells in animals. (2) Cells from mature tissues of adult animals were used rather than embryonic cells as is often done in studies of this type because it is cells of the former type that are most commonly converted to tumor cells in the whole animal. (3) Freshly isolated cells were used rather than established cell lines because many significant changes

may occur in cells as a result of prolonged culture.
(4) A system was used in which virtually all of the
cells in culture are transformed in short periods
of time.

These criteria were largely satisfied by using
pectoral muscle fibroblasts from young adult chickens. The fibroblasts were passaged twice and divide
into two groups. One group of cells was used as
the normal control while the other was transformed
with the Schmidt-Ruppin strain of the Rous sarcoma
virus. When the two groups of cells were grown in
a conventional serum-containing medium with either
physiological concentrations of Ca^{++} or low concentrations of that ion, both normal cells and trans-
formants grew profusely. However, when plasma was
substituted for serum in a low Ca^{++} medium the
transformed cells grew profusely while the normal
cells, although maintained, remained essentially
quiescent. This was true despite the fact that
the normal cells attached firmly to the plastic
culture dishes. It was thus possible to reproduce
in cell culture the situation as it is found to
occur in a host in which the tumor cells proliferate actively while the growth of the normal cells

is precisely regulated. It was found, further, that
when the normal fibroblasts were maintained in an
essentially resting state for three or more days and
then either serum was substituted for plasma or the
concentration of the Ca^{++} ion was raised to physiological levels in the plasma-containing medium, the
normal cells grew profusely. The amount of growth
of the normal cells reflected within limits the
level of the Ca^{++} ion in the culture medium. The
results of these studies indicate, then, that the
proliferation of normal fibroblasts is regulated by
some Ca^{++}-mediated function and that growth of
transformed fibroblasts results either from an increased ability of those cells to take up Ca^{++} from
dilute solution or from an alteration or bypass of
that function (See Fig. 6). These studies showed
further that the Ca^{++} ion functioned by initiating
some critical process in the G_1 phase of the cell
cycle and that, once this function was activated,
it set into operation the necessarily complex
series of reactions that led to chromosomal DNA
replication, mitosis, and finally to cell divisions.
Several important questions remain unanswered. What
is the precise nature of the Ca^{++}-mediated function?

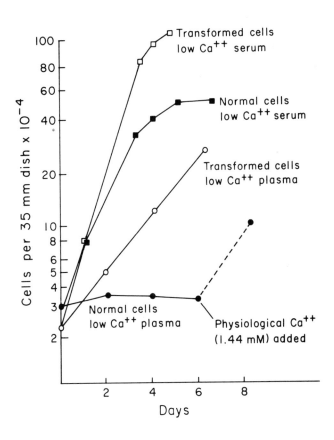

Fig. 6.   Proliferation of normal and Rous sarcoma
virus-transformed chicken fibroblasts cultivated
on a low-calcium medium containing heat-inactivated
chicken plasma or serum prepared from the same lot
of blood. Note the transformed cells proliferate
actively on a low-calcium medium containing either
serum or plasma. The normal cells proliferate
actively on a low-calcium serum-containing medium
but not on a low-calcium plasma medium, where they
are maintained but remain essentially quiescent.
The resting normal cells can be made to proliferate
actively either by adding physiological levels of
calcium to the plasma-containing medium or by sub-
stituting serum for plasma in the low-calcium
medium. Growth of normal cells appears to be regulated by some calcium-mediated function, while
growth autonomy of transformed cells appears to be
largely independent of that function.

Does the mechanism described above apply only to virally transformed chicken fibroblasts or to neoplastic fibroblasts generally? Does it apply to cells other than transformed fibroblasts? The fact that an abundance of evidence now exists to show that Ca^{++} and the principal hormones of the calcium homeostatic systems are major physiological regulators of proliferation of thymic lymphoblasts and bone marrow erythroid cells and perhaps peripheral lymphocytes and liver parenchymal cells suggests that these findings may have broader implications (155). The results of these and similar studies appear to represent a start in the right direction and, if now explored further, should provide meaningful insight into those changes in proliferative behavior that constitute the ultimate basis of the tumor problem.

ABILITY OF CANCER CELLS TO INVADE AND METASTASIZE. In addition to an inability of tumor cells to regulate the mechanisms that normally control cell growth and division, which is a feature common to both benign and malignant tumors, an ability to invade underlying tissues and to detach small

groups of cells from a tumor, which then move to
distant sites through the blood vessels and lymph
channels where new tumors may develop, characterize
the cancerous state. It is well known, however,
that certain normal cells such as the macrophages,
leukocytes and lymphocytes, etc., invade tissues
intensively and move freely through an organism and
thus show certain fundamental attributes of cancer
cells. Such cells do not, however, develop into
tumorous growths because their division mechanism
is precisely regulated. It is possible, moreover,
to cause normal epithelial cells to look and behave
for the time being as though they were cancerous by
treating them with a substance such as Scharlach R
(43). This dye (since shown to be weakly carcinogenic but not acting as a carcinogen in these
studies) causes epithelial cells directly exposed
to it to multiply actively, invade underlying
tissues deeply, and even enter the blood vessels
and lymph channels. Although such epithelial cells
mimic the malignant state perfectly, they revert
completely to normal when the Scharlach R disappear
from the site of injection. These observations
indicate that all of the genetic information neces-

sary to establish the cancer phenotype is present
in normal epithelial cells and the maintenance of
that state is merely a question, as we shall see
later, of how that information is regulated.

The ability of cancer cells to invade and
metastasize appears to reflect changes at the surface of those cells. It has long been recognized
that many animal cancer cells are more easily
separated from one another by mechanical means than
are cells from benign tumors or those of corresponding normal tissues. It has been suggested that
this reduced adhesiveness shown by the cancer cells
constitutes the physical basis of malignancy (27).

In addition to a reduced "stickiness" of the
surfaces of cancer cells, such cells may show differences in movement and behavior from their normal
counterparts when grown in cell culture. Normal
cells such as, for example, fibroblasts when grown
in monolayer culture tend to move and when two or
more cells come in contact with each other they
adhere to one another and cell movement commonly
stops. Such cells line up beautifully in parallel
array. Cancer cells, on the other hand, behave
quite differently. The movement of such cells is

less coordinated, growth is not contact-inhibited,

and the cells move freely over one another and

often pile up in random fashion (See Fig. 7). The

saturation density reached by tumor cells in culture

is commonly greater than that found for normal cells

grown under similar conditions of culture. These

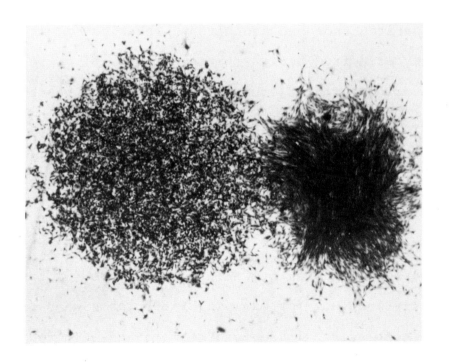

Fig. 7. Left: A colony derived from cloned hamster cells transformed by the Schmidt-Ruppin
strain of the Rous sarcoma virus. Right: A
revertant colony derived from a cloned line of
transformed cells. (Courtesy of Dr. Ian Macpherson)

differences in movement and behavior appear to reflect differences in the surface properties of the
cells.

Alterations in the surface properties of cancer cells are manifested in other ways. Many such
cells clump or agglutinate when treated with spe-
cially prepared plant proteins (lectins) such as
wheat germ agglutinin or concanavalin A, while
similar receptor sites required for agglutination
are exposed only for very short periods in the normal cell cycle in normal cells (22). The receptor
sites in normal cells may be exposed persistently
by treating those cells with a proteolytic enzyme
such as trypsin, thus suggesting that those sites
are covered by a proteinaceous material during most
of the life history of the normal cell while they
are continuously exposed in a transformed cell (23).
Consistent differences were found, moreover, to
exist between binding of the plant lectins and the
normal or tumor phenotype in temperature-sensitive
SV40 transformed 3T3 cells. Thus, when the transformed cells were grown at 32°C and showed the tumor
phenotype, they bound significantly more lectin than
when incubated at 39°C and showed the normal pheno-

type (104). The plant lectins have also been found to be as effective as insulin through direct inter- action with insulin receptors in enhancing the rate of glucose transport as well as in other insulin- mediated responses (31). These studies would sug- gest, then, that alterations in the transformed cell surface detected by the lectins may be involve in the loss of growth control shown by the trans- formed cells.

Although the surface changes as expressed by an increased agglutinability with the plant lectins may or may not in themselves ultimately be found to be related to changes in growth regulation, they may, nevertheless, reflect a series of general mem- brane alterations which could be importantly in- volved in the development of a capacity by tumor cells for autonomous growth, invasion, and metas- tasis.

In animal cancer cells characteristic antigen may be found either within a cell or on the surface of a cell. Those found on the surface, like the receptor sites for the plant lectins, reflect changes in the surface properties of those cells. The surface antigens have been termed transplantation antigens and are particularly interesting because, as we shall see later, they may render tumor cells vulnerable to immunological attack. It has been established, moreover, that transplantation antigens are different and distinct for each individual cancer induced by a chemical carcinogen but they are shared by all cancers induced by the same virus. This finding thus provides one approach for determining whether a tumor of unknown etiology is caused by one or another of the oncogenic viruses.

That specific substances may be determining factors in invasion and metastasis is suggested by recent findings. A migration factor that could contribute importantly to the malignancy of SV28 cells (a line of BHK21/13 hamster cells transformed by the SV40 virus and chosen for its malignancy) has now been demonstrated (24). It was found in those studies that when a monolayer culture of normal Balb/C 3T3 cells is wounded by scraping away part of the cell sheet, the normal cells do not migrate into the cleared area unless serum is present in the culture medium. In contrast, SV40 transformed Balb/C 3T3 cells do migrate into the wounded area in a serum-free medium. A migration factor, which

differs from the serum factor, was found to be
released into a serum-free medium by the highly
malignant SV28 cell line. Although this factor
has not as yet been characterized chemically, the
most purified fractions thus far obtained have
about 1500 times the specific activity of whole
calf serum. What relationship, if any, this factor
has to the so-called "overgrowth stimulating factor"
described above is not as yet known. Should the
elaboration of such a migration factor(s) be found
to be associated with the malignant state in other
systems but not with the normal or benign state it
would, needless to say, have profound implications
as far as our understanding of the ability of cancer
cells to invade and metastasize is concerned.

Very recently it has been reported that a
contact-inhibited melanocyte culture produces a
diffusible protein-containing substance which is
capable of restoring contact inhibition of growth
to highly malignant hamster melanocytes (85).
Thus, both the capacities for migration as well as
for contact inhibition of growth appear, in certain
instances at least, to be controlled by specific
substances.

Functionally, changes in the properties of the membrane systems found in cancer cells result in greater autonomy of such cells in relation to their environment. This is evidenced most clearly by the fact, as we have seen, that virally transformed chicken fibroblasts grow profusely in a selective culture medium that does not support the continued growth of comparable normal cell types. Striking increases in the rate of uptake of certain solutes by virally transformed animal cells have, moreover, been observed by a number of investigators (46, 61, 71). A similar phenomenon, also determined by new membrane properties, has been reported for plant tumor cells (18, 158, 159). In those systems progressive increases in the permeability of the cell membranes to certain inorganic ions and organic solutes have been found to result during the transition from a normal cell to a rapidly growing, fully autonomous tumor cell. The ions were found, moreover, to fully activate a series of biosynthetic systems the products of which are importantly involved in establishing a capacity for autonomous growth in the plant tumor cell.

It has been found, moreover, that a signifi-

cant correlation exists between the level of the
electrical transmembrane potential (E_m) of somatic
cells and the degree of their mitotic activity (28).
Variations in the electrical transmembrane potential are assumed to be the consequence of corresponding shifts in the steady state ionic balance o
the cell, thus implying that the observed mitotic
effects accompanying changes in the electrical
transmembrane potential are mediated through change
in the intracellular levels of specific ions, particularly Na^+ and K^+. These studies place emphasis
on the cell surface because of the central importance of the surface in E_m generation mechanics and
they might ultimately provide important insights
into the function and relationships between alterations in the cell surface following transformation
that commonly lead to excessive division by those
cells and the biophysical properties of the cell
membranes.

   All of these studies indicate that many cellu
lar properties including some of the most important
ones that distinguish normal cells from cancer cell
may be expressed as surface properties and further
studies in this already very active area will doubt

less be most rewarding.

CHAPTER III

ON THE ORIGIN OF THE CANCER CELL: SOMATIC MUTATION

HERITABLE CELLULAR CHANGES THAT UNDERLIE THE TUMOROUS STATE

In any attempt to characterize the nature of the heritable cellular change that underlies the tumorous state, it should be remembered that the genetic material, whether present in the nucleus of a cell or whether introduced by an oncogenic virus, must be implicated either directly or indirectly in controlling cellular metabolism. The pertinent question is not, therefore, whether the genetic material is implicated in the tumor trans-

60

formation, for it clearly is, but rather whether
the heritable cellular change underlying tumorigenesis involves a permanent alteration of a
mutational type or whether it is epigenetic in
nature and is concerned merely with a persistent
change in the expression of that information. This
distinction would appear to be more than just of
academic interest since if it is genetic in nature
it implies irreversibility and is susceptible only
to methods of control presently being applied, e.g.,
surgical removal of the new growth and/or selective
destruction of the tumor by chemicals and radiation.
Ultimately, genetic engineering techniques may be
developed that will permit repair of damage resulting from mutation. If, on the other hand, epigenetic
mechanisms are involved, then the cancerous state
is potentially reversible and, if that concept is
true, opens, in principle at least, entirely new
avenues of approach to the tumor problem.

There are a number of different genetic and
epigenetic mechanisms which could account for the
heritable cellular change that leads to the tumorous
state. Among these might be mentioned (1) changes
in the integrity of the genetic information resulting

from a point mutation(s) or somatic crossing over;
(2) quantitative or qualitative changes in the
balance of chromosomes or chromosome parts due to
nondisjunction, chromosomal rearrangements, poly-
ploidy or aneuploidy; (3) addition of new genetic
information resulting from infection by the oncogenic viruses; or (4) epigenetic modifications
which are concerned not with changes in the integrity of the genetic information present in a cell
but rather with changes in the expression of that
information. The problem thus appears to resolve
itself into learning which one or more, if any, of
the several different genetic or epigenetic changes
listed above is most likely to underlie the tumorous
state generally. What, then, is the evidence that
can be marshalled to support each of these concepts?

SOMATIC MUTATION. The fact that the characteristic
properties of tumor cells, like genetic traits generally, are faithfully transmitted to their descend-
ants over long periods of time has over the past
half century appealed to many as an argument in
favor of the mutation theory of cancer. The fact,
moreover, that oncogens such as ionizing radiations

and carcinogenic chemicals are not only powerful
cancer-producing agents but are also effective mutagens when applied not only to microorganisms but to
certain animal cells in culture appears to provide
further support for proponents of the mutation
theory. It is also true that both radiation and
carcinogenic chemicals affect the genetic material
of a cell. For example, the wave lengths of ultraviolet light that are effective in inducing tumors
are those that are preferentially absorbed by and
that damage the structure of the nucleic acids.
Carcinogenic chemicals are known, moreover, to react
chemically with the nucleic acids and proteins.
Cells treated with either physical or chemical oncogens, whether transformed or not, often show an
abnormal chromosome picture and this is true of most
advanced tumors as well. Finally, in certain rare
instances in which a mutation is known to have
occurred (retinoblastoma) or the chromosome complement of the cells of an individual is abnormal
(Fanconia's anemia, Down's syndrome, etc.), proneness for the development of cancer is heightened
significantly. All of these observations would
appear to provide powerful support for the mutation

theory for the origin of cancer and yet in no
instance has a causal relationship been established.
Let us therefore examine briefly each of the points
raised above to see if acceptable alternatives to
the mutation theory of cancer can be provided.

Ionizing radiations and/or carcinogenic chemicals are now known to cause cancers by at least two
different and distinct mechanisms and possibly a
third other than the postulated somatic mutation.
The first of these is the demonstration that physical and chemical oncogens may activate latent viruses in cells and that it is those viruses that
are, in fact, responsible for the neoplastic transformation. It was believed for many years that
certain leukemias and lymphosarcomas that arose in
mice as a result of whole body X-irradiation of the
animals were the result of somatic mutation. More
recent studies have shown, however, that these
diseases are caused by specific oncogenic viruses
which are present in cells of the mice in a latent
or oncogenically inert state but, following irra-
diation, they become oncogenically active and are
capable of regularly producing leukemias when they
infect appropriate normal non-irradiated cells (84).

A second and quite different example of tumors arising from ionizing radiation and not due to somatic mutation is that which results from a disturbance of growth regulation involving such endocrine glands as the ovaries, the thyroid, and the pituitary. It has been found, for example, that in mice certain tumors (luteomas, granulosa cell tumors) arise with high frequency in the ovaries following exposure of the animals to ionizing radiation (143, page 100). Subsequent studies showed that such tumors could be prevented by shielding one ovary from the source of radiation, by grafting an unirradiated ovary into an animal that had been exposed to radiation, or by the injection of estrogen into an irradiated animal. Further studies disclosed that tumors arose in the irradiated ovaries because of a reduced production of estrogen and this, in turn, led to an increased production of the gonadotropic hormone by the pituitary gland. When this increase in gonadotropin was prevented, tumors did not develop despite the fact that the ovaries had been exposed to the same dose of ionizing radiation that normally induced the formation of tumors. It seems clear, therefore, that ionizing radiation can affect the regulation of growth in such a way that it leads indirectly to the induction of tumors which do not, in these instances, appear to result from somatic mutations.

It has been found, further, that when human skin or hairless mouse skin was exposed to ultraviolet light a compound with known carcinogenic properties, cholesterol-α-oxide, was identified among the photoproducts present in the skin cells (10). This finding suggests that the photochemical conversion of skin cholesterol to an oncogenic substance may play a role in the induction of certain skin cancers and, if true, would provide an alternative mechanism to that postulating damage to the chromosomal DNA by ultraviolet light as a cause of skin cancers. Yet others (26, 124) who have compared the effects on human xeroderma pigmentosum and normal human skin found that damage to chromosomal DNA caused by ultraviolet light in normal cells was quickly repaired while damage in xeroderma pigmentosum was not, and they suggest that such unrepaired damage may be etiologically involved in the inception of the tumors. Which one, if either, of these two mechanisms is involved is not yet known.

One of the most appealing arguments advanced
by proponents of the mutation theory of cancer is
the presumed correlation that exists between muta-
genicity and carcinogenicity among the physical and
chemical oncogens.

As pointed out earlier in this discussion, the
chemical carcinogens include among their numbers
very different types of compounds which appear structurally to have little in common. It has now been
demonstrated, however, that many are similar to one
another in the electronic nature of their ultimate
active forms. They appear to be substances with
electron-deficient atoms which react chemically with
electron-rich atoms such as those found in the DNA's,
RNA's, and proteins. This also appears to be true of
most mutagens. While the chemical mutagens have been
shown to react with the chromosomal DNA to accomplish
their effects, the critical target molecule(s) in a
cell that is affected by the carcinogenic chemicals
has yet to be characterized. Many of the chemical
carcinogens in their ultimate active forms have been
found to be very effective mutagens when applied to
microorganisms in culture. Certain of the carcinogens (for example, the simple alkylating agents) have

been shown to cause base-pair substitutions in the
chromosomal DNA, while many others have been found
to be frame-shift mutagens when applied to microorganisms (2). While the mutations produced in
microorganisms by the chemical carcinogens are of
a random type affecting many different loci, the
cellular transformations resulting from the application of those substances to mammalian cells appear
to result in the same type of heritable cellular
change. Under the best conditions the efficiency
of transformation of mammalian cells in vitro may
approximate 100% of the cell population treated.
Such a frequency of transformation is far higher
than would be expected for randomly occurring mutations. In contrast, when microorganisms are similarly treated with the ultimate active form of a
carcinogen, approximately 10,000 mutations result
under the best conditions at any one locus for
every 100 million cells treated (2). Thus, if
transformation is due to mutation it would be
necessary to postulate the presence in mammalian
cells of some extremely sensitive locus (or loci)
which is regularly affected by a chemical oncogen(s)
and which invariably leads to the development of

the tumorous state. This, if true, would be the
first example of a directed mutation(s) caused by
a specific substance in cells of higher organisms.
In comparing microorganisms and mammalian cells it
must also be recognized that a bacterial genome is
basically haploid while mammalian cells commonly
contain a diploid complement of chromosomes. Thus
a recessive mutation at a single gene locus would
be easily recognizable in a microbial system while
both genic alleles would have to be affected in a
mammalian system for the mutation to be dominant.
These facts make it even more difficult to reconcile
the differences that are found to exist between the
numbers of mutations recorded for bacteria treated
with chemical carcinogens and the high degree of
transformation obtained when mammalian cell systems
are similarly treated.

The results reported above would appear to
be equally consonant with inductive type mechanisms
which clearly do not involve mutations. Thus, although the chemical carcinogens have been shown to
be effective mutagens when applied not only to
microorganisms but to mammalian cells as well, it
does not necessarily follow that transformation to

the tumorous state is the result of somatic mutation at the nuclear gene level.

THE DELETION OF CELLULAR COMPONENTS. The deletion
of cellular constituents and activities which could
be attributable to mutations have been described as
occurring in many different tumors. A particularly
interesting and much studied example of this is
found in the azo dye-induced tumors (hepatomas) of
the liver (97). It was observed in those studies
that livers of rats fed aminoazo dyes contained protein with covalently bonded carcinogen while there
was an almost complete absence of carcinogen-binding
protein once a tumor had developed. This led to the
theory, known as the protein deletion hypothesis,
that carcinogenesis, in these instances at least,
results from a permanent alteration or loss of
protein essential for the regulation of growth.
Subsequent studies (129) showed, moreover, that
most of the bound dye was present in an electro-
phoretically slow moving class of proteins known as
the h2 proteins and that the liver tumors contained
almost none of this class of protein. If, now, the
h2 proteins are growth regulators, as had been

postulated, then it should be possible to inhibit

growth by providing those proteins to the tumor

cells that had lost the ability to synthesize them.

It was, in fact, found that when enriched h2 protein

fractions were added to HeLa cells (tumor cells of

human origin) or L cells (derived from normal mouse

fibroblasts) growth of those cell lines was inhibited.

This inhibition was reversible simply by washing the

cells and thus removing the h2 proteins from the

cultures. An analysis of the h2 protein fraction

showed, however, that the inhibitory substance

present in that fraction was the enzyme arginase

(130). The inhibitory effect of the arginase could

be overcome by supplementing the culture medium with

the essential amino acid arginine. Inhibition thus

resulted simply from a deprivation and ultimate

starvation of the arginine-requiring cell lines.

While it is true that by far the most of the car-

cinogenic azo dyes are bound to the h2 proteins of

the cytoplasm, some binding has also been found to

occur to nuclear protein as well as to the nucleic

acids (114, 151). Which of these bindings is of

central importance to the cellular transformation

and whether a mutation, which may or may not be

etiologically involved, occurs in these systems is
not yet known.

CHROMOSOMAL ABNORMALITIES. Another argument that
proponents of the mutation theory of the origin of
cancer have advanced deals with the great frequency
with which chromosomal abnormalities are associated
with the malignant state. It is, of course, well
known that chromosomal anomalies exist in many advanced tumors and it is often possible to find a
variety of karyotypes within a given tumor. This
finding has led to the suggestion that deviations
from the original diploid karyotype may represent
manifestations of genetic evolution in which the
dominating cell line represents those cells that
are best adapted to their immediate environment.
Thus different karyotypes found within a given
tumor could confer a very real selective advantage
as far as growth of the tumor is concerned (83).
This does not, of course, necessarily mean that
such chromosomal anomalies are the cause of the
tumorous state; they may simply be the result. The
fact, moreover, that a significant number of malignant tumors have now been found that have an essen-

tially normal diploid karyotype indicates that
chromosomal abnormalities need not be involved in
either the establishment or in the maintenance of
the tumorous state. All of this does not, of course,
mean that tumors cannot arise as a result of chromosomal imbalance and this theory is, in fact, favored
in certain quarters at the present time (64). The
chromosomal imbalance theory and its meaning as
far as the etiology of cancer is concerned will be
considered again later in this discussion.

It is, of course, possible that very small
changes may occur in the integrity of the genetic
information present in the nucleus of a cell and
that it is those changes rather than the more crude
shifts in the chromosomal pattern that are involved
in establishing the tumorous state. It has been
reported, for example, that certain mammalian cells,
including hamster cells transformed by the Schmidt-
Ruppin strain of the Rous sarcoma virus, may show
an increased incidence of chromosome breaks and this
appeared to involve specific chromosomes more often
than others. It was suggested as a result of those
findings that the chromosome breaks may be etiologically significant and may act as indicator systems

for point mutations (103). Subsequent studies from
another laboratory dealing with the normalization of
cloned hamster cells transformed with the Schmidt-
Ruppin strain of the Rous sarcoma virus showed,
however, that the reversion from the malignant state
to the normal state appeared to be associated with
the loss of the oncogenic virus by the cells (91)
(See Fig. 7). It thus appears that the observed
chromosomal breaks are not directly concerned with
the basic cellular mechanisms underlying tumorigenesis in this system. The virus itself rather
than mutation resulting from the chromosome breaks
caused by the virus appears, in this instance, to
determine the fate of the cells.

There are a number of different tumors that
arise in individuals all of whose cells are known
to contain mutations or chromosomal abnormalities.
One of the more interesting of these is a rather
rare tumorous disease of the eye known as retinoblastoma. This disease is inherited as a recessive
trait and commonly appears in children who have
inherited a single recessive mutant gene from each
parent. The presence of these recessive genes would
not appear to be the cause of the cancer because

the mutant genes are present in all of the cells
of such an individual and one does not find tumors
developing from the general population of the cells
of those individuals. Instead, only certain specific cells of the eye become converted into tumor
cells. While tumors often arise in both eyes at
about the same time, there are many instances recorded in which a tumor develops in only one of the
eyes despite the fact that the mutant genes are
present in retinal cells of both eyes and those
cells go through precisely the same developmental
stages until the time that the tumor is initiated.
It would thus appear that the immediate cause of
retinoblastoma is not the mutant genes since the
presence of those genes is not in itself sufficient
to cause a tumor to be initiated. The mutant genes
must, nevertheless, play an important role in pre-
disposing certain specific cells of the eye to the
tumor transformation either by rendering such cells
particularly vulnerable to a misprogramming of the
genetic information during a specific stage in
their differentiation or by making certain retinal
cells unusually susceptible to some oncogenic agent.
It is also possible that one or more additional

mutations may occur which render the cells neoplastic (79).

Another example that is often cited and in
which mutation may be involved is found in a human
disease known as chronic myelogenous leukemia. In
this instance a correlation has been found to exist
between the presence of an abnormal chromosome and
the disease. The Philadelphia (Ph[1]) chromosome,
which has lost approximately one-half of its long
arm, is believed to be a highly specific morphological marker for that disease. Recent studies
suggest that the chromosome part is, in fact, not
lost from the cell but is translocated from chromosome 22 (the Philadelphia chromosome) to chromosome
9 and is replicated with that chromosome (115).
This, then, would appear to be a classic example of
somatic mutation involving the permanent rearrangement of the genetic material present in a cell.
Yet it is difficult to know what the correlation
that has been found to exist between the Ph[1] chromosome and the disease really means because (1) the
correlation is not a perfect one since it has been
found to exist only in 85-90% of typical cases
studied (105); (2) the Ph[1] chromosome has been found

in a few individuals who did not develop the disease; and (3) that abnormal chromosome may be present not only in the granulocytes, the cell type
involved in this leukemia, but also in erythrocytic
and megakaryocytic cells all of which probably arise
normally from a common precursor. Yet in the latter
two instances the cells do not commonly replicate
autonomously although they may increase in numbers
above those normally found. It may be noted, moreover, that in the case of chronic myelogenous leukemia it is the stem cells found in the bone marrow
and perhaps the immature granulocytes present in the
blood that proliferate in abnormal numbers. The
progeny of those cells found in the peripheral blood
mature and differentiate and no longer appear capable of autonomous growth despite the fact that they
contain the Ph[1] chromosome. As in the case of
retinoblastoma cited above, the chromosomal defect
observed in chronic myelogenous leukemia could simply predispose the affected cells to some environmental factor which is the real cause of the leukemia. It is well known, for example, that aneuploid cells, which are commonly found in individuals
with Fanconia's anemia, are far more susceptible to

transformation by certain oncogenic viruses (SV40)
than are cells with the normal diploid complement
of chromosomes (141).

The mutation theory of cancer could, theoret-
ically at least, easily account for the origin of
a tumor cell. One would, for example, only have to
postulate the loss through mutation of an appropriate regulatory gene(s) or an inability resulting
from mutation of epithelial cells or certain other
cell types to produce or respond to a chalone to
account for the unrestrained growth of a tumor cell.
It has not as yet been demonstrated experimentally
that the mutation of a regulatory gene(s) or an
inability, as a result of mutation, to synthesize
a chalone leads to the formation of the tumorous
state. Certain cancer cells have, in fact, been
shown to synthesize significant amounts of a chalone
(29, 30). All of this does not necessarily mean
that the tumorous state cannot arise as a result of
somatic mutation at the nuclear gene level. It
simply means that that theory has not as yet been
demonstrated unequivocally for any tumor system
in the vertebrates or for tumors of higher plant
species. It is, nevertheless,.conceivable that a

mutation(s) may have occurred and be implicated
etiologically in some situations but that such a
mutation(s) is expressed and thus recognizable only
under certain very special conditions. Should such
a mutation(s) be found, the mutant gene(s) would
probably act via epigenetic mechanisms to alter the
expression in other parts of the host cell genome.
Perhaps genetic analyses deriving from the newer
methods of somatic cell hybridization will assist
in clarifying this matter.

CHAPTER IV

ADDITION OF NEW GENETIC INFORMATION

THE ONCOGENIC VIRUSES

Are there, then, alternative mechanisms for
which experimental evidence has been provided and
which can account for the origin of a cancer cell?
One such mechanism which is now well established
involves the addition of new genetic information
into a cell as the result of infection by the oncogenic viruses. Although the addition of new
genetic information may involve a change, as does
somatic mutation, in the integrity of the genetic
information present in a cell, it is basically
quite different from mutation and is commonly known
as transformation. In considering the question as
to how new genetic information present in the

oncogenic viruses converts a normal cell into a
tumor cell several possibilities must be considered.
The first of these is that the viral nucleic acids
function as templates for the synthesis of new and
specific substances which, in turn, are responsible
for establishing and maintaining the tumorous state.
Alternatively, new and specific products derived
from the activities of the viral genome may be
exerting their biological effects indirectly by
bringing about a persistent activation of that
segment of the host cell genome that is concerned
with continued cell growth and division. Finally,
the viral nucleic acids may persistently activate
host cell functions by means other than those involving transcription and translation of the viral
genome. In some instances the relation may perhaps
be a purely physical one or, on the other hand,
an oncogenic virus by simply replicating actively
in a cell may produce persistent metabolic changes
that result in the development of the tumorous
state.

THE ONCOGENIC DNA VIRUSES. Among the DNA-containing

viruses that have been shown to be oncogenic are
the polyoma virus, the simian vacuolating virus 40
(SV40), certain of the commonly found adenoviruses,
the Shope papilloma virus, as well as herpes-type
viruses. Of these, herpes-type viruses have been
commonly found associated with and may be etiologically involved, either by themselves or perhaps in
association with oncogenic RNA viruses (82), in
certain human cancers (e.g., lymphomas, cervical
carcinoma, and nasopharyngeal carcinomas) (77). One
of the central problems in cells transformed by any
of the oncogenic viruses is a determination of the
exact form of the association that develops between
the virus and a target host cell. By far the most
thoroughly studied systems as far as host cell-virus
interactions and viral functions are concerned are
those dealing with the very small DNA-containing
viruses, notably polyoma and SV40. The relation of
these viruses to a target cell may be of several
different kinds. In the productive type of infection the virus multiplies essentially unchecked and
eventually lyses and kills a cell. In the second
or abortive type of infection there is little or no
productive infection but, instead, a transformation

leading to the tumorous state. Transformations in
these systems commonly occur with low frequency and
only one to two per cent of the cellular population
is converted into tumor cells following treatment
with the virus. If instead of plating the infected
cells in the usual manner they are suspended in a
viscous solution of methacel, up to half of them
form colonies and behave as though they were tumor
cells. When such colony-forming cells are removed
from the methacel solution and plated in the usual
manner the vast majority revert again to normal cell
types (132). These results were interpreted to mean
that transformation may be either temporary, in
which case the cells again become normal, or permanent if the viral DNA becomes integrated into the
DNA of the genome of the target cell. That integration may occur is now well established and it has
been found that certain transformed cells contain
about 20 SV40 virus DNA equivalents per cell. The
viral DNA molecules are linked to cellular DNA by
alkali-stable covalent linkages (120). Although,
as indicated, no productive infection occurs in
transformed cells, it is possible to rescue the
complete virus from such cells, in certain instances

at least, by fusing the transformed cells with
certain untransformed cell lines, indicating that
all of the genetic information necessary for the
synthesis of the whole virus is present in the
transformed cells (80, 152).

The DNA of these viruses has a molecular
weight of about three million and is of a circular
double-stranded type that contains about 5,000
nucleic acid bases. Since three of these bases are
required to specify one amino acid in a polypeptide
chain, it follows that the 5,000 bases can specify
about 1,700 amino acids. It can be calculated,
moreover, from the molecular weight of the protein
coat of the virus that between one-third and one-
fourth of the genetic information present in the
viral genome is required to specify for viral coat
protein. The remaining genetic information, which
can specify for about 1,200 amino acids, is sufficient to code for between four and eight new proteins depending on their size. These are, therefore
the maximum number of viral genetic functions that
can be involved in the transformation process.

Of the seven viral functions that have thus
far been characterized in these systems two are

particularly suspected as being etiologically involved in the transformation process. The first
and perhaps a highly significant cellular function
identified with viral activity is the activation
of the synthesis of chromosomal DNA and proteins
and the enzymes required for the production of
those substances in an infected cell. It has
been suggested that the viral gene which directly
or indirectly induces cellular DNA synthesis may
be the essential event involved in the transformation process in these systems. A second and
perhaps also important virally specified function
is the presence at the surface of transformed cells
of a new antigen, the transplantation antigen.
This may be important because it may reflect
changes at the surface of transformed cells which
alter the response of those cells to exogenous
regulatory influences.

A third viral function that has been characterized but that does not appear to be relevant to
transformation is a virus-specific intracellular
antigen, the T antigen, which differs in immunological specificity from both the transplantation
antigen and the protein of the viral coat. That

the T antigen may not be necessary and is certainly
not in itself sufficient to maintain the tumorous
state is evidenced by the fact that during the normalization of cells transformed by either the polyoma or SV40 virus the T antigen continues to be
detectable in the cells.

The other four viral functions that have thus
far been characterized appear to be irrelevant to
transformation. Thus the problem appears to be
narrowly restricted to two viral functions, neither
of which can as yet be pointed to with certainty as
far as their significance to the etiology of the
tumor cell transformation is concerned.

Although, as indicated above, the DNA of these
viruses is integrated during transformation into the
chromosomal DNA of the host cells, it has been found
that the transformed state is not necessarily irre-
versibly fixed in transformed cells. It has been
reported, for example, that the progeny of single
cells in which the transformed state had become a
hereditary cellular property produced a high frequency of revertants that showed the normal phenotype (110, 112). This reversion from the tumorous
state to the nontumorous state appeared to be accom-

panied by changes in the normal diploid complement of chromosomes. The reverted cells, which still contained part or all of the virus genome as evidenced by the presence of the T antigen in the cells, appeared to have either somewhat more or somewhat less than the normal diploid number of chromosomes (11).

THE ONCOGENIC RNA VIRUSES. The oncogenic RNA-containing viruses, also known as the leukoviruses, are widely distributed in nature. These are medium-sized viruses that contain a single strand of RNA that has a molecular weight of 10-12 million. The viral nucleic acid component is therefore much larger and can code for a considerably greater number of proteins than can the nucleic acids of the small DNA-containing viruses described above. The RNA viruses have been divided on the basis of their morphology into what are called C-type particles (Rous sarcoma, mouse leukemia and sarcoma viruses, etc.) and B-type particles (mouse and monkey mammary tumor viruses, etc.). Multiplication of these viruses in a host cell does not result in the death of the cell, as is commonly observed with other viruses, but, rather, causes the infected cell to replicate actively. Transformation, of a normal cell into a tumor cell occurs with high efficiency and commonly the entire population of treated cells in culture is transformed into the neoplastic state. The infected cells may or may not produce the complete virus particle but in either case the viral genetic information is passed from one cell generation to the next.

Certain of these leukoviruses may be spread horizontally, that is, by contact with an infected animal. This is true in the case of certain oncogenic viruses in the chicken where contact infection has been convincingly demonstrated. The mammary tumor virus of the mouse is, moreover, commonly transmitted through the mother's milk, thus making breast cancer in this instance a communicable disease (9). Vertical transmission, which refers to the transmission of the virus from parent to offspring through the gametes, is assumed to be the predominant route for naturally occurring leukemia viruses in the mouse. The mouse leukemia virus may be considered to be the prototype of the ubiquitous C-type particles that have now been reported to

exist in many species of animals and have been found
in snakes, chickens, mice, cats, rats, hamsters,
cattle, pigs, monkeys, and perhaps man. These
viruses have been shown to be etiological agents in
naturally occurring cancers in chickens, mice, and
cats and are suspect in many other species of animals including man. The C-type viruses in mice have
been studied in great detail and a new antigen,
the group specific antigen, was found which is
specified by the virus and is common to this whole
group of leukemia and sarcoma-producing viruses.
This new antigen was found not only in mouse leukemia and sarcoma cells, which was to be expected
since such cells were known to contain the viral
genomes, but it was also detected in normal embryonic tissues, but not in adult tissues, of all mouse
strains studied including those believed to be free
of either leukemia or sarcoma viruses. This entirely unexpected finding led conceptually to the
formulation of the oncogene theory of cancer which
states in essence that all adult vertebrates carry
within their cells an unexpressed oncogenic virus
genome and that the difference between those individuals who develop cancer and those who do not

resides simply in whether the oncogene present in
the viral genome is expressed or repressed (68,
139). Since the viral genome is postulated to be
present in cryptic form in all cells of vertebrates
and since it is transmitted from cell to cell as a
characteristic Mendelian trait, its presence in a
cell could no longer be considered abnormal since
it is an intrinsic part of the normal genome of a
cell. Thus the basic cellular mechanism underlying
this type of heritable cellular change would be
epigenetic in nature since, according to this concept, whether or not cancer develops is determined
by whether the oncogene is expressed or repressed.
It should be noted, however, that the oncogene is
only part of the viral genome that is postulated
to be integrated into the genome of a cell. Other
parts of the viral genome specify for the production
of the group specific antigen, the infectious virus,
etc. These several viral functions can be expressed
independently of one another as evidenced, for example, by the fact that the group specific antigen
can be detected in cells in the absence of either
productive viral infection or any evidence of tumori
genesis. This fact has permitted a determination

of the presence of C-type viruses in cells where
their presence had previously not been suspected
and has, in part at least, been responsible for the
suggestion that genomes of these viruses are universally present in cells of vertebrates.

The oncogene theory, if found to be true,
would represent a generalization which could account
for the development of all tumors.   Such cancer-
inducing factors as radiation, carcinogenic chemicals, as well as aging and the hormonal status of
a host would simply be looked upon as being co-
carcinogens that derepress and hence render functional a universally present oncogene.   There is
now an abundance of evidence to show that clonal
lines of mouse, hamster, and rat cells which do not
commonly produce the complete virus can be made to
do so and become transformed when treated with
radiation, chemical carcinogens, and mutagens.

The thymidine analogs 5-bromodeoxyuridine and
5-iododeoxyuridine have also been found to be highly
effective inducers of certain RNA viruses which are
similar to but distinct from the common mouse leukemia virus (89).   Such viruses, called endogenous
viruses, can be induced in all strains of mice thus

far tested and are also found in cells of other
species. Certain strains of mice are known to contain at least three distinct C-type RNA viruses.
One of these is the mouse leukemia virus; the second, which can be induced chemically, replicates
poorly in cultures of mouse cells; while a third
does not replicate in mouse cells and, like the
second, does not produce tumors when injected into
newborn mice. Many of these endogenous viruses do
not replicate in cells of their origin but can be
made to multiply in cells of other species. One
example of this type of virus, which are known as
xenotropic viruses, has been obtained from placental
tissue of a baboon. This C-type virus does not
replicate in cultured placental cells of primates
but can be made to multiply in brain cells of the
dog. Xenotropic viruses have not been shown to be
oncogenic in any species although some viral onco-
logists feel that they may somehow be implicated
in the etiology of certain tumors. The evidence,
nevertheless, suggests that C-type RNA-virus genetic
information may be present but unexpressed in cells
of many different species of animals.

The oncogene theory can be and has recently

been put to experimental test with the use of two
pairs of identical human twins (7). One member of
each pair was afflicted with acute myelocytic leukemia while the other member showed no evidence of
the disease. If the oncogene theory is correct,
then one should find in these instances identical
DNA sequences in the diseased and healthy member of
each twin pair since the methods used in this study
detected all gene sequences whether active or
silent. The results of this study showed, however,
that unique leukemia-specific DNA sequences were
present in the diseased member of each twin pair
and absent in the healthy member. These data imply
that the additional specific leukemic information
must have been inserted into the DNA of the host
cell subsequent to fertilization and thus argues in
this instance against the oncogene theory which
postulates vertical transmission through the germ
line of the oncogene. Since the specific leukemia
sequences are inserted after fertilization, the
authors believe that their findings are more consistent with the provirus theory of oncogenesis
(135).

    According to the provirus hypothesis, the

genetic information present in the oncogenic RNA
viruses is transcribed via an RNA-DNA hybrid into
a double stranded DNA molecule which, after being
integrated into the chromosomal DNA of a target
cell, may function as a template for the synthesis
of viral RNA molecules. This theory received
strong support with the isolation and characterization of a new type of enzyme, an RNA-dependent
DNA polymerase commonly known as reverse transcrip-
tase, which translates RNA into DNA (4, 138). This
enzyme has been found to be associated with all
RNA-containing cancer-producing viruses and with
only a very few viruses not known to cause cancer
(e.g., visna virus and simian foamy virus are not
known to be oncogenic in animals). That an integration of provirus DNA into the host cell DNA
occurs now appears well established in the Rous
system (145).

The oncogene theory and the provirus theory
are similar in that both postulate a double stranded
DNA intermediate form which is integrated into the
chromosomal DNA of the host cell and which replicates with that DNA. These two theories differ from
one another in that the oncogene theory postulates

that the viral genetic information was integrated into the chromosomal DNA at some earlier period in evolution and has persisted as an intrinsic part of that DNA in cells of all vertebrates. The provirus theory postulates, on the other hand, that the new viral genetic information present in a transformed cell is derived as the result of recent infection by an exogenous oncogenic virus.

A second, more recent theory, the protovirus hypothesis, proposes apparent vertical transmission of information for cancer even though the germ line does not contain the required genetic information either on its chromosomes or in the form of the complete virus. According to this hypothesis, which is described in detail elsewhere (137), the germ line is postulated to contain only the potential for genetic evolution by somatic cells of the information required for cancer formation. This information is believed to arise de novo as a result of multiple cycles of DNA→RNA→DNA information transfer either within a cell or between cells. It has been suggested that the protovirus hypothesis may apply to normal developmental processes as well as to tumorigenesis.

The discovery of temperature-sensitive mutants of the Rous sarcoma virus has permitted the development of experimental systems that lend themselves admirably to meaningful studies of many kinds. When, for example, chick fibroblasts are infected with a thermostable mutant of the Rous sarcoma virus, the cells are transformed into tumor cells when incubated at a temperature of $36^{\circ}C$ (permissive temperature) but appear normal by all criteria when those same infected cells are cultured at $41^{\circ}C$ (nonpermissive temperature). Infectious virus is produced by the cells equally well at both temperatures. The temperature-sensitive process is completely and repeatedly reversible in both directions. Controlled systems of this type are extremely useful because they permit a characterization of specific cellular changes that are strictly correlated with and/or etiologically involved in the transformation process. These studies clearly demonstrate, further, that the genetic information present in an infected cell and that leads to the tumor phenotype can be readily manipulated in these systems leading to cells that show the normal phenotype (131, 142, 150, 156).

That a normalization of the tumorous state may, in fact, occur with the use of Rous sarcoma virus-infected hamster cells has been demonstrated (91) (See Fig. 7). In those studies cloned lines of cells in which the transformed state had become an hereditary cellular property were plated out periodically and it was shown that a significant number of progeny of the transformed hamster cells recover from the tumorous state and appear normal in every respect. Under the best conditions it was reported such transformed populations of cells showed a percentage of revertant colonies that increased from 19% after three weeks in culture to 98% after eight weeks passage in culture. Such rates of reversion are not observed when chicken cells are similarly transformed by the Rous sarcoma virus. Reversion in the case of the transformed hamster cells resulted either from the loss of the viral genome by those cells or from the fact that the viral genetic information was present but was completely repressed. In either case, the results of this study suggest that a functional viral genome is essential for the maintenance of the neoplastic state in the Rous system.

CHAPTER V

EPIGENETIC CHANGES

CANCER AS A PROBLEM IN DEVELOPMENT

Very commonly found examples of heritable cellular changes that are basically different from both somatic mutation and cellular transformations that follow infection by the oncogenic viruses are the changes that accompany cell differentiation during the normal course of development. This type of heritable cellular change is epigenetic in nature and is concerned with persistent changes in the expression of the genetic information that is present in the nucleus of a cell. It is now believed that more than 90% of the genetic information found in the nucleus of cells of higher organisms is

98

repressed and hence nonfunctional and that different
genes or constellations of genes are responsive to
different specific signals that derepress them and
regulate their activities. Thus differences among
cells with an identical complement of genes are
believed to be due to the activity of different
genes in different kinds of cells. With a model
such as this it is easy to understand why, for example, nucleated red cells synthesize hemoglobin
while the white blood cells do not, why kidney cells
produce L-amino oxidase while liver cells do not
but, instead, synthesize as a product of their
differentiation serum albumin. A persistently
dividing cell such as a tumor cell produces, on the
other hand, significant amounts of a specialized
protein in the form of microtubules which has a
highly specialized function to perform during mitosis. Variable gene activity against a constant
cellular genome is, then, the guiding concept upon
which much of the current research in the field of
normal cellular differentiation is directed. Can
this concept be applied to the cancer problem? Is
cancer simply a problem of anomalous differentiation
in that the basic cellular mechanisms that underlie

normal cellular differentiation and tumorigenesis
are fundamentally similar?

Before considering this matter it should be
noted that cellular differentiation, like the neoplastic transformation, represents a highly stable
heritable change and in extreme cases of terminal
differentiation (e.g., mature red blood cells of
mammals and lens fiber cells which have lost their
nuclei) is clearly irreversible. Even the relatively undifferentiated stem cells of the various
tissues from which tumors commonly arise are strongly determined for the cell type into which they
ultimately differentiate. Thus although such cells
contain a complete complement of genes, they are
programmed for particular patterns of metabolism
which are strongly fixed in such cells and are not
easily manipulated. It would, therefore, only be
in the more favorable situations that a reversal of
the tumorous state would be expected to be demon-
strable even though the potential for reversibility
might be present in tumor cells of many different
kinds. It should perhaps also be mentioned here
that a reversal of the tumorous state does not
necessarily mean reversion to the normal state.

It should be recalled that many secondary changes
such as, for example, chromosomal anomalies, alterations in respiration, deletion of enzymes, etc.,
may and commonly do occur in certain tumors. Thus
even if those properties of a cell that lead to
autonomous growth were potentially reversible, the
result would not necessarily be a normal cell since
the recovered cell might retain the secondarily
acquired properties originally possessed by the
tumor cell. Even though such a reverted cell would
be abnormal it would, nevertheless, be nontumorous
and thus fulfill the criteria for the reversion
from the malignant to the nonmalignant state.

In order to test the concept of the reversibility of the tumorous state experimentally it would
appear necessary to demonstrate that the genomes of
normal and tumor cells are genetically equivalent.
This could perhaps be accomplished most convincingly
by demonstrating that the tumorous state is a
reversible process and thus showing that a persistent change in the integrity of the genetic information present in the nucleus of a cell is not an
essential prerequisite for either the establishment
or the maintenance of the tumorous state. That a

normalization of tumorous growth may, in fact, occur
has now been well documented in a wide spectrum of
organisms ranging from tumors found in higher plant
species to those present in man. Selected examples
of the type that best illustrate this phenomenon
will be described below.

REVERSAL OF THE TUMOROUS STATE IN PLANTS. The
first reported attempts to convert tumor cells of
a transplantable type into normal cells were those
carried out with the use of plant tumor systems.
These studies were successful largely because of
two properties that are characteristic of higher
plant species. The first of these is the unique
manner in which dicotyledonous plants grow. Primary
growth in such species results from the very rapid
division, subsequent elongation, and finally differentiation of meristematic cells at the extreme
apex of a shoot or a root. A second property that
proved useful in demonstrating the reversibility
of the tumorous state is that somatic cells of
higher plants may be totipotential. The progeny
of single somatic cells are capable of developing
into normal, fully fertile plants. By combining

these two characteristics it has now been possible
to achieve the normalization of tumor cells in three
different and quite distinct plant neoplasms.

1. The crown gall disease. The typical crown gall
tumor cell is characterized by powers for rapid proliferation, limited capacities for differentiation,
and tissue composed of such cells lacks an ability
to organize structures such as roots or leaves. It
was found, however, that if totipotential cells were
transformed to a moderate degree there was produced,
in place of the characteristic crown gall tumor, a
complex overgrowth, or teratoma (12). This new
growth was characteristically composed of a chaotic
assembly of tissues and organs that showed varying
degrees of morphological development. When sterile
tissues from the morphologically abnormal but organized structures found on the teratomas were isolated
and planted on a simple, selective culture medium
the teratoma cells grew profusely and indefinitely,
as did the characteristic crown gall tumor cells,
on the medium that did not support continued growth
of normal cells. The teratoma cells differed from
the typical crown gall tumor cells in that they

retained indefinitely in culture a capacity to
organize tumor buds and shoots. When such tumor
shoots from cloned teratoma cell lines were isolated
and forced into very rapid but organized growth as
a result of a series of tip graftings to morphologically distinguishable, healthy varieties of the same
species, they gradually recovered from the tumorous
state and some ultimately flowered and set fertile
seed (16). The results of these studies clearly
show that the nuclei of the normal cells and of the
tumor cells are genetically equivalent, suggesting
that we are dealing here with differences in the
expression of the genetic information in the normal
and tumor phenotype rather than with changes involving the deletion or permanent rearrangement of the
genetic information present in those cells.

Subsequent studies showed that not only teratomas but perhaps typical crown gall tumors as well
may recover from the tumorous state (119). A typical unorganized but uncloned tumor cell line that
had been carried continuously in culture more than
15 years was used in those studies. This tumor line
had never shown the slightest tendency to organize
either roots or shoots during its prolonged growth

in culture. It was found, however, that if that
tissue was placed on a special inductive culture
medium, shoots could be made to organize. Such
shoots were isolated and some were made to root.
The rooted shoots were then planted in soil where
they grew and some of the plants flowered. None of
these plants were completely normal in appearance.
A chromosomal analysis of the plants showed that
all contained an abnormal complement of chromosomes
and some were clearly aneuploid. Two points of
interest emerge from this study. The first of these
is that the tumor cells had retained during their
prolonged period in culture the potentialities to
organize shoots and that those potentialities were
never expressed unless the tumor cells were placed
under very special environmental conditions. The
second point of interest is that, despite the fact
that the plants that developed from the tumor tissue
often showed a highly abnormal chromosome picture
and were abonormal in appearance, they, nevertheless,
had recovered from the tumorous state.

2. Kostoff genetic tumors. A second nonself-
limiting neoplastic disease of plants in which a

recovery from the tumorous state has now been
demonstrated involves genetic tumors that arise
regularly and spontaneously in certain interspecific
hybrids in the genus Nicotiana (128). When two
plant species such as, for example, Nicotiana glauca
(2n = 24) and Nicotiana langsdorffii (2n = 18) are
crossed and the seed of the F_1 hybrid (2n = 21) sown
the resulting plants commonly develop normally during the period of their active growth and in the
absence of irritation. Once the plants reach maturity, however, a profusion of tumors arise spontaneously on all parts of the hybrid (See Fig. 8).
When the tumor cells are isolated and planted on a
simple, chemically defined culture medium they grow
profusely and indefinitely on that medium that does
not support the growth of normal cells from either
parent. In a most interesting recently published
experiment differentiated leaf cells from the two
parent species were isolated and grown in culture.
The cell walls were removed enzymatically and the
resulting protoplasts were mixed together and hy-
bridized in culture (25). Where successful fusion
of the protoplasts was achieved the amphiploid hybrid cells (2n = 42 fertile) grew on a simple cul-

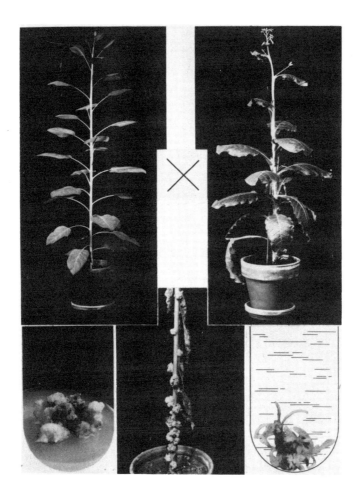

Fig. 8. Kostoff genetic tumors of plants. Upper:
parental species: (Left) Nicotiana glauca (2n = 24);
(Right) Nicotiana langsdorffii (2n = 18). Below:
(Center) Fl hybrid (2n = 21). When the hybrid
reaches maturity a profusion of tumors invariably
develops from all parts of the plant. When mature
differentiated leaf cells from both parents are
isolated and fused in culture the resulting amphiploid (2n = 42) is tumorous but can be made to
recover from the tumorous state and produce plants
that set fertile seed. Thus, despite serious
chromosomal imbalance, the same abnormal karyotype
can give rise to neoplastic growths, on the one
hand, and to normal-appearing plants, the cells of
which are differentiated and fully functional.

ture medium while the unfused cells or fused cells
of either parent did not. The hybrid cells were
thus behaving in culture like the tumor cells in
that they grew profusely on a culture medium that
did not support the growth of fused cells of either
parent. When these hybrid cells were cultured further they organized tumor shoots, and when those
shoots were tip-grafted to appropriate stock plants
they grew in an organized manner and not only ultimately flowered and set fertile seed but developed
spontaneous tumors at the graft union.

This experimental test system is particularly
illuminating because it clearly demonstrates that,
despite a serious chromosomal imbalance in all of
the cells of the hybrid plant, that same abnormal
karyotype can give rise, on the one hand, to a morphologically normal-appearing plant all the cells
of which are beautifully differentiated and are
fully functional. That same abnormal karyotype can,
on the other hand, give rise to neoplastic growths.
These two metastable states are readily reversible
in both directions under defined experimental conditions.

The genetic tumors in plants may be considered

to provide a model for the so-called chromosomal imbalance theory of cancer which postulates that tumors arise because of an upset in the balance between those genes that determine growth and those that are concerned with the regulation of growth (11). The findings reported above, which demonstrate that despite serious chromosomal imbalance the tumorous state is completely reversible, would appear significant and to provide strong support for the concept that the neoplastic state, like normal development processes, may stem from persistent changes in the expression of a genetically equivalent genome.

3. Habituation. When normal plant cells are grown in culture for prolonged periods of time they may acquire, as do animal cells, neoplastic properties. In the plant systems these result from the acquisition by the cultured cells of a capacity to synthesize persistently the two growth-regulating substances, essential metabolites, and vitamins that the cells at the time of their isolation from a plant did not possess. The biosynthetic systems shown to be newly activated may become unblocked either individually or more than one, or all, may

become activated more or less simultaneously. When

the two growth-regulating systems, the auxins and the

cell division factors, which, it will be recalled,

establish the pattern of metabolism concerned

with cell growth and division together with those

required to permit that pattern to be expressed, are

all persistently activated, then the cells behave

like typical plant tumor cells in that they grow

profusely in culture on a minimal medium and when

implanted into an appropriate host, develop into

typical tumors. Once these essential biosynthetic

systems are activated in a cell the newly acquired

capacities may be retained indefinitely by those

cells. This, then, is a heritable cellular change

that is highly stable, occurs in the absence of any

recognizable oncogen, and is very similar to that

resulting from the tumor transformation in the crown

gall disease. This phenomenon is known in the plant

field as habituation. Of particular interest in

this connection is a preliminary report which indi-

cates that habituation for a single factor, in this

instance the cell division-promoting factor, occurs

with a frequency of between two and three orders of

magnitude greater than that found for spontaneously

occurring random mutations (8).

That habituation is completely reversible with the use of techniques described above has now been demonstrated with the use of a significant number of cloned lines of habituated tissues (8, 90). Since this phenomenon is completely and regularly reversible the results of these studies provide the ultimate proof that the tumorous state may arise and be perpetuated as a result of persistent changes in gene expression. In the case of habituation nothing has been added, deleted or rearranged. Thus we see that all of the genetic information necessary to account for the establishment and maintenance of the neoplastic state is present in the normal cell genome and since this process is regularly reversible one does not have to postulate drastic changes of a mutational type to account for the continued abnormal and autonomous proliferation of a tumor cell. Any new genetic information that is added to a cell as a result of infection by an oncogenic virus might perhaps be looked upon as somehow persistently activating that segment of the host cell genome that is concerned with continued cell growth and division rather than coding specifically for one or more substances that are required for the autonomous proliferation of tumor cells.

These plant tumor systems provide the best evidence yet available to indicate that the tumor problem may be in essence a problem of anomalous differentiation and that the basic cellular mechanisms underlying the tumor transformation and normal cellular differentiation may, in fact, be similar. Both appear to depend for their expression on the selective activation and repression of genes.

REVERSAL OF THE TUMOROUS STATE IN ANIMALS. 1. Lucké adenocarcinoma of the frog. The question that arises next is whether a reversal of the tumorous state is unique to plant tumor systems or whether it has, in fact, broader biological implications. A most remarkable example of this in the animal field is provided by work carried out on the Lucké adenocarcinoma of the leopard frog. This is a highly malignant tumor that is caused by a herpes-type virus (102). The virus in this instance rather specifically transforms the convoluted tubules of the kidney. An attempt was made in these studies to determine the developmental potentialities of a

cancer nucleus. In order to have a nuclear marker
to distinguish cancer nuclei from normal nuclei,
adenocarcinomas were induced in a triploid line of
frogs and the nuclei of the resulting cancer cells
had a triploid complement of chromosomes (96).
Nuclei from these triploid tumors were then isolated
and implanted into activated but enucleated normal
frog eggs. It was found in those studies that not
only did the cancer nuclei participate in normal
cleavage but a significant number of apparently
normal, fully functional triploid tadpoles were
obtained (See Fig. 9). The results of these studies
are of considerable significance as far as the biology of cancer is concerned. Most striking perhaps
was the absence of any evidence of malignancy in
the tadpoles that had developed from a cancerous
nucleus. When those nuclei were placed in the
proper cytoplasmic environment the cells were no
longer capable of unrestrained growth but rather
responded beautifully to the cellular mechanisms
that normally control cell differentiation and
organogenesis. The cancer nucleus was thus effectively domesticated by those cytoplasmic factors
that regulate nuclear gene activity during the nor-

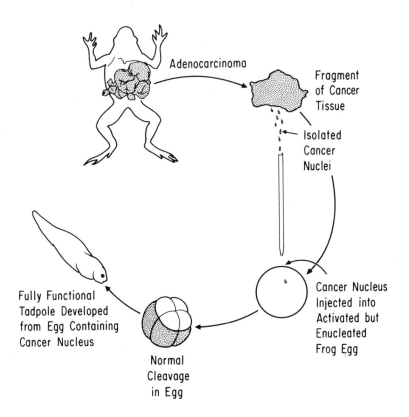

Fig. 9. Diagram showing the fate of a nucleus
from a malignant Lucké adenocarcinoma cell when
implanted into an activated but enucleated normal frog egg. Note normal cleavage occurs and
apparently normal, fully functional tadpoles
develop from cells containing cancer-derived
nuclei. These studies suggest in the strongest
manner that the normal egg cytoplasm is capable
of reprogramming the genetic information present
in the cancer nucleus in such a way as to permit
normal development to proceed.

mal course of development. This study clearly

demonstrates that what a nucleus, whether normal

or cancerous, does is determined largely by the

cytoplasmic environment in which that nucleus is

found. A true understanding of the cancer problem

may therefore have to await very precise knowledge

of the cytoplasmic factors and mechanisms that are

so intimately concerned with both the regulation

of the cell division process and with cell differen-

tiation that occur during the normal course of

development (14, See chapter 5).

2. Teratocarcinoma of the mouse. The examples of

a reversal of the neoplastic state described thus

far have all dealt with lower forms of life, and

it might well be argued by some that what happens

in plants and lower vertebrates has little relevance

to mammalian oncology. What, then, do we know

about the occurrence of this phenomenon in mammals.

Three examples of this type will be discussed

briefly because they illustrate quite admirably the

principles involved in the normalization of a cancer

cell. The first of these is a malignant teratocarci-

noma of the mouse. This is a rather rare tumor that

contains derivatives of all three embryonic germ
layers, and from eight to fourteen very well differentiated cell types (epithelial cells, nerve
cells, bone, cartilage and muscle cells, tooth buds
hair follicles, etc.) are scattered in completely
disorganized array in the tumor. Interspersed amon
these well differentiated cell types are essentiall
undifferentiated cells which are known as embryonal
carcinoma cells. When such a tumor is transplanted
serially from mouse to mouse this broad spectrum of
cell types is reproduced indefinitely. The questio
that arose in studying this tumor was whether the
differentiated cells developed independently or
whether they all arose from a common precursor or
stem cell. To test that latter hypothesis experimentally, single embryonal carcinoma cells were
injected into the peritoneal cavities of mice (78).
In all of the more than 40 instances in which the
single cells established themselves and grew, malig
nant tumors developed that killed the animals in a
few weeks time. A histological study of those
tumors showed that they were composed of a typical
mixture of eight to fourteen different, well
differentiated cell types together with embryonal

carcinoma cells. The differentiated cell types
were found to have lost their malignant properties.
These studies clearly demonstrate, then, that the
embryonal carcinoma cell is a multipotential cell
which is malignant in the undifferentiated state
but which is capable of giving rise to a broad
spectrum of differentiated derivatives that have
lost their malignant properties. It should be noted,
however, that cellular differentiation in itself
does not always terminate the malignant character.
Certain cell types (parietal yolk sac carcinomas
and choriocarcinomas) derived by differentiation
from stem cells of teratocarcinomas retain their
malignant properties.

3. The epidermoid (squamous) carcinoma in animals
and man. The teratocarcinoma is, as indicated, a
rather rare tumor, so let us look next at a much
more commonly found cancer, the epidermoid (squamous)
carcinoma. This type of tumor is derived from the
basal cells of the skin or of the hair follicles
and may be initiated by either ionizing radiation
or carcinogenic chemicals. It is well known that
when a normal basal cell divides it gives rise to

one derivative that differentiates and becomes
heavily keratinized to form the keratinized epi-
thelium, while the other member of the pair retains
the potentialities of the basal cell from which it
was derived.

The epidermoid carcinoma typically consists
of an agglomeration of so-called epidermal cell pegs
which are embedded in a matrix of normal connective
tissue. Division occurs only among those cells that
form the rim of each peg while the entire interior
of a peg is composed of cells that have differentiated and have become heavily keratinized. The
differentiated cells often show pycnotic nuclei
and appear to have reached the end of the line as
far as further growth is concerned (See Fig. 10, B)
A study was undertaken to determine the origin of
the differentiated cells at the center of a peg and
it was found that they were derived from the dividing cancer cells at the rim of each peg (109). It
was found, further, that when the dividing cancer
cells were implanted into appropriate hosts they
gave rise to typical epidermoid (squamous) carcinomas while when the differentiated cells at the
center of a peg were similarly implanted tumors did

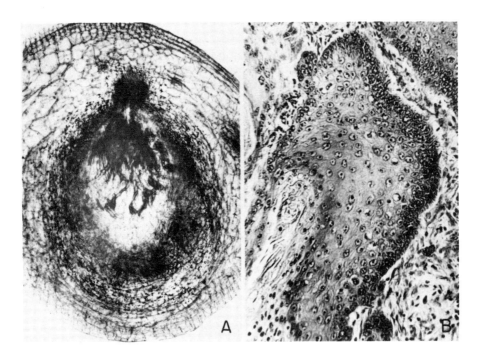

Fig. 10. Histological sections of: A, a small
secondary tumor of the sunflower; and B, epidermoid (squamous) carcinoma of a rat. Note that
between 1/3 and 1/2 of the central core of the
tumor in A is composed of tracheary elements that
had undergone terminal differentiation and death.
The entire central core of the peg shown in B is
composed of keratinized cells that were derived
from the dividing cancer cells at the rim of the
peg and that had undergone terminal differentiation with the loss of neoplastic properties.
(Courtesy of Dr. Roy E. Albert)

not develop. Thus the cancer cell is behaving like
the normal basal cell in that when it divides it
gives rise to one derivative that differentiates
and, in this instance, loses its cancerous properties, while the other member of the pair behaves
like the basal cell from which it was derived.
Here, then, is another example of a cancer cell in
a mammal that retains the potentialities for terminal differentiation with the loss of malignant
properties. That most tumor cells retain potentialities for differentiation is evidenced by the fact
that they are classified by pathologists on the
basis of the cell type of their origin and must
therefore show a sufficient capacity for differentiated function to be so classified.

REVERSAL OF THE MALIGNANT STATE IN HUMANS. 1.
Neuroblastomas. The clinical evidence for the spontaneous regression of malignant tumors in man is
now considerable (38). Although many of these
regressions are attributable to immune reactions or
hormonal influences, there are now a significant
number of well documented instances in which such
regressions involve a maturation and differentiation

of cancer cells into cells that have lost their
malignant properties. Interesting examples of
this are found in the neuroblastomas of man. The
neuroblastoma is a highly malignant tumor that is
derived during organogenesis from the primitive
sympathetic nerve cell, the neuroblast. This disease is commonly diagnosed early in life, metastases
soon develop, and in the vast majority of patients
there is a rapid downhill course culminating in
death in a relatively few months. There are dramatic and well documented exceptions to this, however,
in which all of the cells of advanced metastasizing
neuroblastomas matured and differentiated spontaneously into ganglion cells that had lost their malignant properties (32, 36, 38, 147). Patients in
whom such regressions occurred lived for many years
without recurrence of the malignant tumor.

SUBSTANCES THAT REGULATE THE CANCER PHENOTYPE. It
has, moreover, now been possible to cause neuroblastoma cells to differentiate into ganglion-like
cells under defined conditions of cell culture with
the use of a naturally occurring substance, the
nerve growth factor (55). A factor released in

culture from glial cells has also been found to
induce a high degree of morphological differentiation in neuroblastoma cells grown under physiological conditions of culture (101). Here, then, is a
highly malignant tumor of man the cells of which
retain the potentialities for differentiation with
an accompanying loss of their cancerous properties.

Another interesting example of a naturally
occurring substance that can, in this instance,
remove the block for differentiation that is found
in acute myelogenous leukemia of humans is the so-
called MGI protein (40). This differentiation-
inducing protein, which is released in culture by
various normal cell types including spleen, can
cause myeloid leukemic cells to develop into mature
macrophages and granulocytes. The induction of
differentiation in this instance does not require
the addition of adenine or an adenine-containing
co-factor that has been found to be necessary for
the differentiation of normal haematopoietic cells,
since the leukemic cells themselves were found to
produce the required co-factor. Of interest was
the finding that differentiation could be induced
in cloned lines of leukemic cells that no longer

contained a diploid complement of chromosomes (41).
Since the induction of differentiation could be
accomplished in vitro in leukemic cells obtained
from patients with acute myeloid leukemia, it was
suggested that treatment of such patients with the
MGI protein may be of potential value for therapy
of that leukemia (40).

It is clear, therefore, that in both the animal and plant fields tumor cells may retain the
potentialities for differentiation with the loss of
tumorous properties. The problem of control would
thus appear to resolve itself into learning how to
bring about the controlled expression of those potentialities in all cells of a tumor. This, in turn,
would require an ability to manipulate nuclear gene
function at will. There is certainly now no good
reason for believing that nuclear gene function is
beyond hope of correction. We have seen a striking
example in the case of the Lucké adenocarcinoma in
which the activity of the genes in a cancer cell
nucleus, when placed in an appropriate cytoplasmic
environment, was reprogrammed in such a way as to
permit normal development to proceed. Clearly,
these as yet largely uncharacterized cytoplasmic

factors are capable of reprogramming the genetic

information present in the nucleus of a cancer cell.

An understanding of the nature of those factors and

the cellular mechanisms involved in their regulation

would appear to be a first but most important step

to understanding the cancer problem. It has now,

in fact, been possible to reprogram the genetic in-

formation present in certain plant cells in such a

way that it leads to the terminal differentiation

and resulting death of those cells (6). These stud-

ies, which were carried out under precisely defined

experimental conditions, suggest that cyclic 3':5'-

AMP is somehow importantly involved in this type of

cytodifferentiation. Fig. 10, A illustrates this

type of terminal differentiation as it is found in

a young secondary tumor of the sunflower, while

Fig. 10, B shows an example of what appears to be

an entirely analogous situation in the animal tumor

field. In the plant tumor, between one-third and

one-half of the central core of the tumor is com-

posed of highly lignified tumor cells that have

become terminally differentiated into tracheary

elements and have lost, as a result of differentia-

tion, their neoplastic properties. Fig. 10, B

shows a peg of an epidermoid (squamous) carcinoma of the rat in which the entire center of the peg is composed of heavily keratinized cells that were derived from the dividing tumor cells at the rim of the peg and that had lost their malignant properties. Here, then, are two striking examples in which terminal differentiation with the loss of tumorous properties is a characteristic feature of the new growths. The potentialities for terminal differentiation are clearly present in all cells of such tumors and an understanding of the substances and mechanisms that are involved in reprogramming the genetic information present in the tumor cells might well lead to the effective control of such tumors.

A partial or even the very occasional complete self-healing of certain malignant tumors in animals and man is not, moreover, an uncommon observation in general pathology. Since this sort of thing occurs spontaneously, as we know it does in the case of the malignant metastasizing neuroblastomas described above, there is every reason to believe that if the mechanisms underlying such regressions were understood they could be effectively applied as control measures.

In addition to such naturally occurring factors as the MGI protein, the nerve growth factor, and the glial cell factor mentioned above, certain non-naturally occurring substances as dimethyl sulfoxide (DMSO) and 5-bromodeoxyuridine (BdUR) have been found to be effective in redirecting cellular metabolism from that characteristic of the tumor phenotype to that found in the normal phenotype. When, for example, DMSO is applied to erythroid leukemia cells in culture it causes those cells to mature, differentiate and behave in every respect as do comparable normal cell types in vitro (48). Similarly, when highly malignant melanoma cells of the mouse are exposed to BdUR in culture they behave as do normal cells. The point of interest that emerges from this study is that whether the cancer phenotype or the normal phenotype is expressed is determined entirely by whether or not BdUR is present in the culture medium (127). Studies of the type described above demonstrate that nuclear gene function in a cancer cell is not beyond hope of correction, as was believed for so many years, and continued efforts to characterize

more precisely the substances and mechanisms underlying the regulation of nuclear gene activity could
be most rewarding.

A relatively recent and promising approach
to the question of the suppression of malignant
behavior in advanced cancer cell lines comes from
studies on the fusion of normal cells with tumor
cells. Although many studies (5, 33, 117, 121, 126)
had indicated that when normal cells and tumor cells
were fused the tumor character was dominant in the
progeny of the hybrid cell, other studies have indicated that when three different and distinct malignant mouse tumor cell lines were fused with cells
of an essentially normal mouse L-cell line, the
tumor character was largely suppressed (60). Similar results were obtained with hybrids between other
tumor and normal cells (157). That this suppression
of malignancy was, in the first instance, due to
some contribution made by the chromosomes of the
normal cell line is indicated by the fact that this
contribution is lost and the cells again regain
their malignant properties when certain chromosomes
of the normal line are eliminated from the progeny
of the hybrid cells. Since the factor(s) responsi-

ble for the suppression of malignancy in these systems has its orgin on one or more of the chromosomes of the normal cell line it should be possible to map that chromosome(s), locate the position of the effective gene(s), and most importantly, characterize the tumor-suppressing factor itself. If this could be successfully achieved it might provide a useful approach to tumor therapy since a naturally occurring tumor-suppressing factor is involved here.

CHAPTER VI

BIOLOGICAL APPROACHES TO CONTROL

Many experimental approaches based on a knowledge of the biology of cancer and, more particularly, on certain characteristics and requirements that distinguish cancer cells from normal cells have been applied in an effort to control the disease. A few of the more interesting examples of this type will be briefly described.

DIFFERENCES BETWEEN NORMAL AND TUMOR CELLS
THAT MAY BE EXPLOITED THERAPEUTICALLY

BIOCHEMICAL APPROACHES. Extensive comparative biochemical studies of normal and tumor cells have defined differences some of which can be exploited

therapeutically. One significant difference found

to exist between most normal and most tumor cells

was first reported by Otto Warburg in 1923 (148).

This investigator found that the cancer cells with

which he worked characteristically showed aerobic

glycolysis with the production of lactic acid, while

the respiration of comparable normal cells was of

the conventional type. These studies have been

confirmed by others many times and a correlation

has been found to exist between the rate of growth

of different tumor cell lines and the degree of

aerobic glycolysis that those lines show. Such

findings led Warburg to suggest that cancer arises

as a result of irreversible damage to the normal

respiratory system with a switch to glycolytic

pathways that would be required for survival of

the cells (149). More recent studies carried out

with Morris minimal deviation hepatomas have shown,

however, that the more slowly growing of these,

although transplantable and malignant, show little

or no aerobic glycolysis. Aerobic glycolysis also

appears to be a characteristic feature of certain

normal cells, particularly some found in embryos.

The evidence now available suggests that the
aerobic glycolysis found to characterize many
cancer cells is probably a result rather than the
primary cause of the neoplastic state (153). There
have, nevertheless, been attempts made to influence
the respiratory behavior of tumor cells and thus
control tumor development. One interesting example
of this is found in the case of the Plummer-Vinson
syndrome which represents an early stage in the
development of certain cancers of the esophagus and
pharynx. It has been reported that if the diet of
individuals suffering from this condition is heavily
supplemented with nicotinamide, flavin, and salts
of iron, which serve as coenzymes for the normal
respiratory enzymes, the disease can not only be
cured in its earliest stages but perhaps even prevented if the coenzymes are administered at an
early enough time.

Another example in which differences between
normal and tumor cells can be exploited therapeutically is found in certain leukemias and lymphosarcomas, the cells of which possess an absolute exogenous requirement for L-asparagine for their growth.
Most normal cell types are able to synthesize that

compound and, hence, do not require an exogenous source of it. It was found that by introducing into the blood stream of leukemic patients the enzyme L-asparaginase, which destroys free L-asparagine in the body fluids, dramatic remissions were obtained in patients with L-asparagine-dependent leukemias (19). In many instances, however, some leukemic cells remained that did not share this asparagine dependence and as those cells multiplied this form of therapy became inadequate. This system, nevertheless, represents a model and if other differences between normal and tumor cells are found that are perhaps closer to the transformation process itself than is asparagine dependence, they may be more profitably exploited therapeutically.

METHODS FOR PREVENTING THE ACTION OF CHEMICAL CARCINOGENS. Since man living in an urban industrial society is continually subjected to environmental carcinogens, studies are now underway either to attempt to prevent the conversion of such cancer-producing substances into their ultimate active form or to trap the active form after it is produced in a target cell and thus render it harmless. It

has been found, for example, that the inhibitor
7,8-benzoflavone of the enzyme aryl hydrocarbon
hydroxylase, when applied to mouse skin together
with the carcinogen 7,12-dimethylbenz(a)pyrene,
markedly retards the initiation of tumors (76).   It
is known, moreover, that the carcinogenic
N-2-fluorenylacetamide must be converted by the
enzyme sulfotransferase to its strongly electrophilic sulfate ester to be effective in eliciting
the formation of tumors.   It has been reported that
a significant inhibition of liver tumors by that
carcinogen can be achieved by a depletion of the
sulfate pool in cells of test organisms (154).

It has been postulated that because of the
strongly electrophilic nature of the ultimate active
form of many carcinogens it might be possible to
retard or inhibit tumorigenesis entirely by flooding
target cells with strong nucleophiles, thus trapping
the active carcinogen before it binds to the critical macromolecules in those cells.   Some preliminary
data designed to test this hypothesis has shown that
a partial inhibition of liver tumor initiation can,
in fact, be achieved with the use of excess dietary
methionine, cystine, or tryptophan (98).   It has

been suggested, moreover, that such a mechanism
may provide natural protection against the relatively small amounts of environmental carcinogens
likely to be encountered at any particular time.

IMMUNOLOGICAL APPROACHES. A further and most
important difference between cancer and normal cells
is found in the new antigens that are present at
the surface of the tumor cells. Since these new
antigens are different from those exposed at the
surface of normal cells, they are often recognized
by the immune system of an animal as being foreign
substances and thus, as in the case of any foreign
protein, elicit specific immune responses from a
host. There is now considerable evidence to suggest
that these immune responses represent fairly effective defense mechanisms that keep many early cancers
in check and certain of the rather rare instances
of spontaneous regressions of advanced cancers have
been attributed to them. The importance of the
immune response in controlling cancer is evidenced
further by the finding that individuals with primary immunodeficiency diseases (e.g., sex-linked
agammaglobulinemia, IgA deficiency, ataxia-

telangiectasia, Wiskott-Aldrich syndrome, etc.)

have a significantly higher than normal risk of

developing cancers. This fact has been attributed

to deficiencies in the immunologic surveillance

mechanisms found in individuals afflicted with those

disorders.

The functions of the immune defense system

are carried out chiefly by three types of white

blood cells: (1) the plasma cell which produces

specific antibodies against foreign proteins. These

antibodies are released from the cells and circulate

freely in the blood stream and other body fluids.

(2) The cell-mediated immune responses in which

thymus or T-lymphocytes and, to a lesser extent,

the macrophages play an essential role. The

T-lymphocytes are capable of being sensitized to

an antigen and, once sensitized, are capable of

recognizing that antigen and of transferring that

information to other lymphocytes in some as yet

unknown manner. In this way it is possible to

mobilize an immune response on a very large scale

when that is required. In the case of the cell-

mediated immune response the recognition system

remains in the lymphocytes and those cells carry

the attack to the tumor cells where they may cause
a killing of those cells or their rejection from a
host. The sensitized lymphocytes constitute the
main immunological defense against cancer cells.
(3) The macrophages recognize cancer cells and
other foreign substances through what is known as
the recognition factor. This substance has been
found to be an alphaglobulin and may be present in
serum. An inverse relationship has, in fact, been
found to exist between the amount of recognition
factor present in serum and the extent to which a
cancer has developed in a host. It is believed
that a complexing of the recognition factor with
tumor cells is the first step required for destruction of those cells by the macrophages. The failure
of the recognition system would, on the other hand,
permit cancer cells to go unrecognized by the macrophages and thus escape destruction by those cells.

Why, then, if cancer cells are antigenic and
behave as foreign bodies are they not completely
destroyed by the immune response of a host? There
are a number of possible reasons for this. Such
conditions as aging or any one of a number of other
known factors that suppress the normal immune

response could and doubtless do play an important
role in determining whether or not a given tumor
will develop. One form of immunosuppression, which
is known as immunological tolerance, is found to
occur when an animal is exposed to an antigen very
early in life before the immune system has fully
developed. Under these conditions, which is well
illustrated in the case of certain vertically transmitted oncogenic mouse and chicken viruses, the
animals in later life are tolerant to those viruses
and even when large amounts of fully antigenic virus
particles are injected into such animals antibodies
do not form and the animals are incapable of immune
defense against them. This would be a particularly
important consideration if certain human tumors were
found to be caused by vertically transmitted viruses.

Another disturbing consideration is the finding that there may be blocking factors present in
serum that actually protect cancer cells from the
lymphocytes. The thymic lymphocyte-mediated immune
response against tumors may thus be diminished or
even abolished by such blocking factors. Although
earlier studies suggested that the blocking factor
was the specific antibody, more recent investiga-

tions indicate that that factor is either the tumor antigen itself or a complex of the tumor antigen with its specific antibody. It has been suggested that the complexes of antigen with antibody bind to the tumor cells through the antibody moiety and thus prevent recognition of the tumor cells by the thymic lymphocytes.

There is a further problem and that is one concerned with immunoselection. As in any dividing population of cells, when a tumor grows the cells that comprise the new growth often show variations and some of the cells may be more antigenic than others. It is the least antigenic ones that would be expected to survive, and such a selection process might well account for the poor antigenicity shown by many advanced cancers.

Finally, the inadequacy of the immune response is demonstrated further when a host is confronted with a rapidly growing tumor. Although the immune response of the host does not keep such tumors in check, it has been found that when those tumors are excised surgically, the animals resist reimplantation of their own tumor cells. These results suggest that the immune system is, in fact, functional in these animals but is overwhelmed by too great a challenge provided by the primary tumor. There is, moreover, some evidence to suggest that a weak immune response such as might be expected during the earliest stages of tumor growth stimulates rather than inhibits growth of the tumor cells.

Despite these difficulties, tumor immunology offers a promising approach for the control of cancer and methods are now being developed (1) to modify the surface of cancer cells by a variety of means to increase its immunogenicity, and (2) to increase the immune response of a host with the use of immunoadjuvants. The immunoadjuvants most commonly used are of a nonspecific type involving bacteria or bacterial or fungal products. For example, BCG, which is an attenuated form of the tubercle bacillus, has been used clinically and some dramatic remissions have been reported for several types of tumors. The specific mechanisms by which these nonspecific immunoadjuvants stimulate local and general immunological reactivity is as yet poorly understood and the entire problem of immune enhancement is clearly an important area for future study.

The new and distinctive antigens found in cancer cells may be placed in essentially three categories: (1) the surface antigens which are involved in the immune response; (2) the intracellular antigens; and (3) the so-called fetal antigens, which are secreted by the cancer cells and which may be present in the blood of patients having particular types of cancer. The first of these fetal antigens is the carcinoembryonic antigen which is often found in patients with cancer of the colon, rectum, pancreas, and certain other organs. However, this antigen is sometimes found in the absence of tumors, particularly in the case of inflammatory or regenerative disorders. A second fetal antigen is the so-called alphafeto protein which is present in patients having liver tumors (hepatomas) or embryonal carcinomas, while a third fetal antigen is a fetal gastric sulphoglycoprotein which is found in the gastric juice not only in 96% of patients with gastric carcinomas but in 14% of patients with peptic ulcers as well. All three types of fetal antigens are also found in embryonic or fetal tissues but are not commonly present in adult normal tissues, suggesting that the genetic information

coding for these antigens is functional in the
developing embryo but is repressed during late
stages of development and is again expressed during tumorigenesis. These fetal antigens can and
doubtless will be made to serve as important diag-
nostic tools for the presence of otherwise undetect-
able cancer. For a more detailed discussion of the
relationships between immunity and malignancy, the
reader is referred to the following articles (51,
56, 62, 81, 106).

INTERFERONS. A group of naturally occurring substances, known collectively as interferons, has
been found to have profound effects not only
in preventing the transformation process in certain
virally initiated tumors but in arresting progres-
sions as well as in causing regressions in certain
advanced tumors in mice. The interferons, which
are small protein molecules, were initially found
to be produced by and released from cells infected
with a virus. These substances diffuse to neighboring cells and protect those cells not only from
the virus initially involved in establishing the
infection but from other kinds of viruses as well.

It is now believed that viral infections generally
are held in check as a result of this special
defense mechanism. The interferons represent a
group of species-specific substances since, for
example, the interferon that is produced in mouse
cells in response to viral infection, while pro-
tecting other mouse cells, will not protect cells
of other animal species from viral infection. This
same specificity resides in interferons obtained
from human and other animal species. The interferon
response differs from other immune responses in
that the interferons protect cells rather specifically against foreign nucleic acids rather than
against foreign proteins.

The interferons are essentially nontoxic substances and are tolerated by animals in large doses.
In those instances in which advanced tumors of mice
were shown to regress as a result of treatment with
interferon it appeared that the interferon selec-
tively destroyed the cancer cells, which were the
ones that contained the viral genetic information,
without having any effect on the normal noninfected
cells. It was found, however, that as a result of
the sudden killing and massive lysis of the cancer

cells, toxic symptoms developed which, in turn, killed the experimental animals. These toxic effects resulting from cell lysis would appear to be an important consideration when methods dealing with the elimination of massive advanced cancers are being discussed. This sort of thing would not be encountered if cancer cells could be made to differentiate and lose their neoplastic properties, as in the case of the neuroblastomas described above, rather than being killed and lysed by anti-cancer agents.

Studies with the use of interferons as anti-cancer agents are, nevertheless, promising. They have in the past unfortunately been hampered by an inability to obtain sufficient amounts of them for extensive clinical trials. Since these compounds are small proteins this difficulty should be re-solvable in the not too distant future by isolating them, determining their amino acid sequences, and synthesizing them in the laboratory. For a detailed recent account of the interferons the reader is referred to reference 42.

THE CHALONES. The chalones, as indicated earlier

in this discussion, are a group of naturally
occurring substances that are synthesized by cells
and that appear to be importantly involved in the
regulation of the cell division process as well as
in differentiation of such normal cell types as
epidermal cells, liver and kidney cells, granulocytes, as well as certain other cell types (67,
134). Since the antimitotic effect of these substances is tissue specific and since they are
essentially nontoxic they would appear to represent
an almost ideal group of substances for use in the
suppression of growth of those tumors that have lost
an ability to synthesize their own chalones but
remain sensitive to their inhibitory effects. Although these substances are being actively studied
in a number of laboratories and some success in
tumor suppression has been claimed (20, 21, 100),
a great deal more work will have to be done with
them before a critical evaluation of their effec-
tiveness can be made.

OTHER STRATEGIES BEING ATTEMPTED. Since surgery
and other forms of therapy are now quite effective
in dealing with many primary tumors an important

area for study would appear to be the development
of methods for keeping a cancer localized and thus
preventing its dissemination throughout a host.
Several different types of experimental approaches
are now being investigated in an attempt to accomplish this. One of the more interesting of these
attempts is to prevent growth of a primary tumor by
limiting its blood supply. It has long been known
that there exist in malignant tumors normal blood
vessels that supply the tumor with nutrients and
oxygen and that remove metabolic wastes from the
new growth. These blood vessels are essential for
the continued development of the tumor and, if de-
prived of their normal blood supply, the tumors
remain localized in their growth while still very
small. It has recently been found that the tumor
cells themselves produce a specific inducing substance that is diffusible and which when applied
under the skin of mammals induces in a few days an
intricate network of blood vessels (45). This substance is known as the tumor angiogenesis factor
and it appears to be a ribonucleoprotein. It is
clear, therefore, that if ways could be found to
effectively neutralize that substance, growth of

the malignant tumors would remain localized and could be more easily dealt with (44).

A second approach that is now being actively pursued in the laboratory is one involving the use of specific chemicals which have been found in animal experimentation to be more effective in preventing metastases than in inhibiting growth of a primary tumor.

For a summary statement of other new and novel approaches to cancer therapy that are now being attempted, the reader is referred to the material presented in reference 70.

These, then, are some of the more promising areas for study that have resulted from our present understanding of not only the biology of cancer but of the larger problem that is concerned with the factors and mechanisms that are involved in the regulation of normal cell growth and development. It seems rather unlikely at this point that a sing major breakthrough will occur in the immediate future that will eliminate cancer as a major medical problem. The difficulties of dealing with that complex disease must not be underestimated. Signi icant progress has, nevertheless, been made during

the past decade or two and we now appear to be at
the beginning of an understanding of that problem.
As more knowledge is acquired, more fruitful
approaches than are now available will doubtless
suggest themselves and some of these may well prove
successful.

148

REFERENCES

1. Abelev, G. I., Perova, S. D., Khramkova, N. I.,
   Postnikova, Z. A., and Irlin, I. S. Embryonic
   serum alpha-globulin and its synthesis by
   transplantable mouse hepatomas. Biokhimiya
   28:625-634. 1963.
2. Ames, B. N., Durston, W. E., Yamasaki, E., and
   Lee, F. D. Carcinogens are mutagens: a simple
   test system combining liver homogenates for
   activation and bacteria for detection. Proc.
   Nat. Acad. Sci. U.S. 70:2281-2285. 1973.
3. Balk, S. D., Whitfield, J. F., Youdale, T., and
   Braun, A. C. Roles of calcium, serum, plasma,
   and folic acid in the control of proliferation
   of normal and Rous sarcoma virus-infected
   chicken fibroblasts. Proc. Nat. Acad. Sci.
   U.S. 70:675-679. 1973.
4. Baltimore, D. RNA-dependent DNA polymerase in
   virions of RNA tumour viruses. Nature 226:
   1209-1211. 1970.
5. Barski, G., Sorieul, S., and Cornefert, F.
   Production dans des cultures in vitro de deux
   souches cellulaires en association, de cellule
   de caractère "hybride." C. r. Acad. Sci.,
   Paris 251:1825-1827. 1960.
6. Basile, D. V., Wood, H. N., and Braun, A. C.
   Programming of cells for death under defined
   experimental conditions: Relevance to the
   tumor problem. Proc. Nat. Acad. Sci. U.S.
   70:3055-3059. 1973.
7. Baxt, W., Yates, J. W., Wallace, H. J., Jr.,
   Holland, J. F., and Spiegelman, S. Leukemia-
   specific DNA sequences in leukocytes of the
   leukemic member of identical twins. Proc.
   Nat. Acad. Sci. U.S. 70:2629-2632. 1973.
8. Binns, A., and Meins, F., Jr. Habituation of
   tobacco pith cells for factors promoting cell
   division is heritable and potentially reversible. Proc. Nat. Acad. Sci. U.S. 70:2660-
   2662. 1973.
9. Bittner, J. J. The milk-influence of breast
   tumors in mice. Science 95:462-463. 1942.

10. Black, H. S., and Douglas, D. R. A model system for the evaluation of the role of cholesterol α-oxide in ultraviolet carcinogenesis. Cancer Res. 32:2630-2632. 1972.

11. Bloch-Shtacher, N., Rabinowitz, Z., and Sachs, L. Chromosomal mechanism for the induction of reversion in transformed cells. Internat. J. Cancer 9:632-640. 1972.

12. Braun, A. C. Bacterial and host factors concerned in determining tumor morphology in crown gall. Botan. Gaz. 114:363-371. 1953.

13. Braun, A. C. A physiological basis for autonomous growth of the crown-gall tumor cell. Proc. Nat. Acad. Sci. U.S. 44:344-349. 1958.

14. Braun, A. C. The Cancer Problem; A Critical Analysis and Modern Synthesis. 209 p. Columbia Univ. Press, New York and London, 1969. (see Chapter 5)

15. Braun, A. C., Guest Editor. Plant Tumor Research. 235 p. S. Karger, Basel, 1972. (Progr. Exp. Tumor Res., vol. 15)

16. Braun, A. C. The cell cycle and tumorigenesis in plants. in The Cell Cycle and Cell Differentiation (J. Reinert et al., eds.), Springer, Berlin, in press, 1974.

17. Braun, A. C., and Naf, U. A non-auxinic growth-promoting factor present in crown gall tumor tissue. Proc. Soc. Exp. Biol. Med. 86:212-214. 1954.

18. Braun, A. C., and Wood, H. N. On the activation of certain essential biosynthetic systems in cells of Vinca rosea L. Proc. Nat. Acad. Sci. U.S. 48:1776-1782. 1962.

19. Broome, J. D. Evidence that the L-asparaginase activity of guinea pig serum is responsible for its antilymphoma effects. Nature 191:1114-1115. 1961.

20. Bullough, W. S., and Laurence, E. B. Tissue homeostasis in adult mammals. in Advances in Biology of Skin, vol. VII, "Carcinogenesis" (W. Montagna and R. L. Dobson, eds.) chap. 1, p. 1-36. Pergamon Press, London and New York, 1966.

21. Bullough, W. S., and Laurence, E. B. Control of mitosis in mouse and hamster melanomata by means of the melanocyte chalone. European J. Cancer 4:607-615. 1968.

150

22. Burger, M. M. Surface changes in transformed cells detected by lectins. Fed. Proc. 32:91-101. 1973.
23. Burger, M. M., and Noonan, K. D. Restoration of normal growth by covering of agglutinin sites on tumour cell surface. Nature 228: 512-515. 1970.
24. Bürk, R. R. A factor from a transformed cell line that affects cell migration. Proc. Nat. Acad. Sci. U.S. 70:369-372. 1973.
25. Carlson, P. S., Smith, H. H., and Dearing, R. D. Parasexual interspecific plant hybridization. Proc. Nat. Acad. Sci. U.S. 69: 2292-2294. 1972.
26. Cleaver, J. E., and Trosko, J. E. Absence of excision of ultraviolet-induced cyclobutane dimers in xeroderma pigmentosum. Photochem. Photobiol. 11:547-550. 1970.
27. Coman, D. R. Decreased mutual adhesiveness, a property of cells from squamous cell carcinomas. Cancer Res. 4:625-629. 1944.
28. Cone, Clarence D., Jr. Unified theory on the basic mechanism of normal mitotic control and oncogenesis. J. Theoret. Biol. 30:151-181. 1971.
29. Craddock, C. G., Jr. The physiology of granulocytic cells in normal and leukemic states. Am. J. Med. 28:711-725. 1960.
30. Craddock, C. G. The production, utilization and destruction of white blood cells. in Progress in Hematology (L. M. Tocantins, ed.) vol. 3, p. 92-104. Grune & Stratton, New York, 1962.
31. Cuatrecasas, P., and Tell, G. P. E. Insulin-like activity of concanavalin A and wheat germ agglutinin -- direct interactions with insulin receptors. Proc. Nat. Acad. Sci. U.S. 70:485-489. 1973.
32. Cushing, H., and Wolbach, S. B. The transformation of a malignant paravertebral sympathicoblastoma into a benign ganglioneuroma. Am. J. Pathol. 3:203-216. 1927.
33. Defendi, V., Ephrussi, B., Koprowski, H., and Yoshida, M. C. Properties of hybrids between polyoma-transformed and normal mouse cells. Proc. Nat. Acad. Sci. U.S. 57:299-305. 1967

34. Dulak, N. C., and Temin, H. M. A partially purified polypeptide fraction from rat liver cell conditioned medium with multiplication-stimulating activity for embryo fibroblasts. J. Cell. Physiol. 81:153-160. 1973.

35. Dulak, N. C., and Temin, H. M. Multiplication-stimulating activity for chicken embryo fibroblasts from rat liver cell conditioned medium: a family of small polypeptides. J. Cell. Physiol. 81:161-170. 1973.

36. Dyke, P. C., and Mulkey, D. A. Maturation of ganglioneuroblastoma to ganglioneuroma. Cancer 20:1343-1349. 1967.

37. Earle, W. R., and Nettleship, A. Production of malignancy in vitro. V. Results of injections of cultures into mice. J. Nat. Cancer Inst. 4:213-227. 1943.

38. Everson, T. C., and Cole, W. H. Spontaneous Regression of Cancer. 560 pp. W. B. Saunders, Phila. & London, 1966.

39. Faiman, C., Colwell, J. A., Ryan, R. J., Hershman, J. M., and Shields, T. W. Gonadotropin secretion from a bronchogenic carcinoma. Demonstration by radioimmunoassay. New England J. Med. 277:1395-1399. 1967.

40. Fibach, E., Landau, T., and Sachs, L. Normal differentiation of myeloid leukaemic cells induced by a differentiation-inducing protein. Nature New Biol. 237:276-278. 1972.

41. Fibach, E., Hayashi, M., and Sachs, L. Control of normal differentiation of myeloid leukemic cells to macrophages and granulocytes. Proc. Nat. Acad. Sci. U.S. 70:343-346. 1973.

42. Finter, N. B., ed. Interferons and Interferon Inducers. rev. ed. 598 pp. American Elsevier Publ. Co., New York, 1973. (Frontiers of Biology, vol. 2)

43. Fischer, B. Die experimentelle Erzeugung atypischer Epithelwucherungen und die Entstehung bösartiger Geschwulste. Münch. Med. Wchnschr. 53:2041-2047. 1906.

44. Folkman, J. Tumor angiogenesis: therapeutic implications. New England J. Med. 285:1182-1186. 1971.

45. Folkman, J., Merler, E., Abernathy, C., and Williams, G. Isolation of a tumor factor responsible for angiogenesis. J. Exp. Med.

133:275-288. 1971.

46. Foster, D. O., and Pardee, A. B. Transport of amino acids by confluent and nonconfluent 3T3 and polyoma virus-transformed 3T3 cells growing on glass cover slips. J. Biol. Chem. 244:2675-2681. 1969.

47. Foulds, L. Tumour progression and neoplastic development. in Cellular Control Mechanisms and Cancer (P. Emmelot and O. Mühlbock, eds.) p. 242-258. Elsevier Publ., Amsterdam, London, New York, 1964.

48. Friend, C., Scher, W., Holland, J. G., and Sato, T. Hemoglobin synthesis in murine virus-induced leukemic cells in vitro: Stimulation of erythroid differentiation by dimethyl sulfoxide. Proc. Nat. Acad. Sci. U.S. 68:378-382. 1971.

49. Gellhorn, A. Ectopic hormone production in cancer and its implication for basic research on abnormal growth. Advan. Internal Med. 15:299-316. 1969.

50. Gey, G. O. Cytological and cultural observations on transplantable rat sarcomata produced by the inoculation of altered normal cells maintained in continuous culture. Cancer Res. 1:737. 1941.

51. Gold, P. The role of immunology in human cancer research. Canad. Med. Assoc. J. 103: 1043-1051. 1970.

52. Gold, P., and Freedman, S. O. Demonstration of tumor-specific antigens in human colonic carcinomata by immunological tolerance and absorption techniques. J. Exp. Med. 121: 439-462. 1965.

53. Gold, P., and Freedman, S. O. Specific carcinoembryonic antigens of the human digestive system. J. Exp. Med. 122:467-481. 1965.

54. Goldblatt, M. W., and Goldblatt, J. Occupational carcinogenesis. in Industrial Medicine and Hygiene (E. R. A. Merewether, ed.) Part I vol. 3, chap. 3. Butterworth, London, 1956.

55. Goldstein, M. N. Growth and differentiation of normal and malignant sympathetic neurons in vitro. in Cell Differentiation (R. Harris P. Allin, and D. Viza, eds.), p. 131-137. Munksgaard, Copenhagen, 1972.

56. Good, R. A. Relations between immunity and malignancy. Proc. Nat. Acad. Sci. U.S. 69: 1026-1032. 1972.
57. Gordon, M. A genetic concept for the origin of melanomas. Ann. New York Acad. Sci. 71: 1213-1222. 1958.
58. Gospodarowicz, D. Localisation of a fibroblast growth factor and its effect alone and with hydrocortisone on 3T3 cell growth. Nature 249:123-127. 1974.
59. Hamperl, H. Ueber die Entwicklung ("Progression") von Tumoren. Wien. Klin. Wchnschr. 69:201-205. 1957.
60. Harris, H., Miller, O. J., Klein, G., Worst, P., and Tachibana, T. Suppression of malignancy by cell fusion. Nature 223:363-368. 1969.
61. Hatanaka, M., and Hanafusa, H. Analysis of a functional change in membrane in the process of cell transformation by Rous sarcoma virus; alteration in the characteristics of sugar transport. Virology 41:647-652. 1970.
62. Hersh, E. M., Gutterman, J. U., and Mavligit, G. Immunotherapy of cancer in man. 141 pp. C. C. Thomas, Springfield, Ill., 1973.
63. Hieger, I. One in Six: An Outline of the Cancer Problem. Chap. II. 80 pp. Allan Wingate, London, 1955.
64. Hitotsumachi, S., Rabinowitz, Z., and Sachs, L. Chromosomal control of chemical carcinogenesis. Internat. J. Cancer 9:305-315. 1972.
65. Holley, R. W., and Kiernan, J. A. "Contact inhibition" of cell division in 3T3 cells. Proc. Nat. Acad. Sci. U.S. 60:300-304. 1968.
66. Hondius Boldingh, W., and Laurence, E. B. Extraction, purification and preliminary characterisation of the epidermal chalone: a tissue specific mitotic inhibitor obtained from vertebrate skin. European J. Biochem. 5:191-198. 1968.
67. Houck, J. C., and Hennings, H. Chalones; specific endogenous mitotic inhibitors. FEBS Letters 32:1-8. 1973.
68. Huebner, R. J., and Todaro, G. J. Oncogenes of RNA tumor viruses as determinants of cancer. Proc. Nat. Acad. Sci. U.S. 64:1087-1094. 1969.

154

69. Hunter, D. The Diseases of Occupations. 4th ed. 1259 pp. English Univ. Press, London, 1969.
70. Intra-Science Research Symposium, 7th, Santa Monica, 1973. New ideas in cancer chemotherapy; highlights. 49 p. Intra-Science Research Foundation, Santa Monica, 1973.
71. Isselbacher, K. J. Increased uptake of amino acids and 2-deoxy-D-glucose by virus-transformed cells in culture. Proc. Nat. Acad. Sci. U.S. 69:585-589. 1972.
72. Jablonski, J. R., and Skoog, F. Cell enlargement and cell division in excised tobacco pith tissue. Physiol. Plantarum 7:16-24. 1954.
73. Johnson, R., Guderian, R. H., Eden, F., Chilton M.-D., Gordon, M. P., and Nester, E. W. Detection and quantitation of octopine in normal plant tissue and in crown gall tumors. Proc. Nat. Acad. Sci. U.S. 71:536-539. 1974.
74. Kellermann, G., Luyten-Kellermann, M., and Shaw, C. R. Presence and induction of epoxide hydrase in cultured human leukocytes. Biochem. Biophys. Res. Comm. 52:712-716. 197.
75. Kellermann, G., Shaw, C. R., and Luyten-Kellermann, M. Aryl hydrocarbon hydroxylase inducibility and bronchogenic carcinoma. New England J. Med. 289:934- 937. 1973.
76. Kinoshita, N., and Gelboin, H. V. Aryl hydrocarbon hydroxylase and polycyclic hydrocarbon tumorigenesis: effect of the enzyme inhibitor 7,8-benzoflavone on tumorigenesis and macromolecule binding. Proc. Nat. Acad. Sci. U.S. 69:824-828. 1972.
77. Klein, G. Herpesviruses and oncogenesis. Proc Nat. Acad. Sci. U.S. 69:1056-1064. 1972.
78. Kleinsmith, L. J., and Pierce, G. B., Jr. Multipotentiality of single embryonal carcinoma cells. Cancer Res. 24:1544-1551. 1964.
79. Knudson, A. G., Jr. Mutation and cancer: statistical study of retinoblastoma. Proc. Nat. Acad. Sci. U.S. 68:820-823. 1971.
80. Koprowski, H., Jensen, F. C., and Steplewski, Z. Activation of production of infectious tumor virus SV40 in heterokaryon cultures. Proc. Nat. Acad. Sci. U.S. 58:127-133. 1967.

81. Kreider, J. W., and Bartlett, G. L. Recent advances in human tumor immunology. I, II. Penna. Med. vol. 75, Nov. p. 58; Dec. p. 25, 1972.
82. Kufe, D., Magrath, I. T., Ziegler, J. L., and Spiegelman, S. Burkitt's tumors contain particles encapsulating RNA-instructed DNA polymerase and high molecular weight virus-related RNA. Proc. Nat. Acad. Sci. U.S. 70:737-741. 1973.
83. Levan, A. Some current problems of cancer cytogenetics. Hereditas 57:343-355. 1967.
84. Lieberman, M., and Kaplan, H. S. Leukemogenic activity of filtrates from radiation-induced lymphoid tumors of mice. Science 130:387-388. 1959.
85. Lipkin, G., and Knecht, M. E. A diffusible factor restoring contact inhibition of growth to malignant melanocytes. Proc. Nat. Acad. Sci. U.S. 71:849-853. 1974.
86. Lipsett, M. B., Odell, W. D., Rosenberg, L. E., and Waldmann, T. A. Humoral syndromes associated with nonendocrine tumors. Ann. Internal Med. 61:733-756. 1964.
87. Little, C. C. Hybridization and tumor formation in mice. Proc. Nat. Acad. Sci. U.S. 25:452-455. 1939.
88. Little, C. C. The genetics of cancer in mice. Biol. Rev. Cambridge Phil. Soc. 22:315-343. 1947.
89. Lowy, D. R., Rowe, W. P., Teich, N., and Hartley, J. W. Murine leukemia virus: high-frequency activation in vitro by 5-iododeoxyuridine and 5-bromodeoxyuridine. Science 174:155-156. 1971.
90. Lutz, A. Morphogenetic aptitudes of tissue cultures of unicellular origin. in "Colloq. Internat. Centre Nat. Recherche Sci. (Paris), No. 193, Les Cultures de Tissus de Plantes; (Proc. 2nd Internat. Conf. Plant Tissue Culture, Strasbourg, France, July 6-10, 1970)" pp. 163-168. Paris, Centre National de la Recherche Scientifique, 1971.
91. Macpherson, I. Reversion in hamster cells transformed by Rous sarcoma virus. Science 148:1731-1733. 1965.

92. Marks, L. J., Russfield, A. B., and Rosenbaum, D. L. Corticotropin-secreting carcinoma. J. Am. Med. Assoc. 183: No. 2, 115-117. 1963.
93. Maugh, T. H., II. Chemical carcinogenesis: a long-neglected field blossoms. Science 183: 940-944. 1974.
94. Mazia, D. Mitosis and the physiology of cell division. in The Cell (J. Brachet and A. E. Mirsky, eds.) vol. 3, p. 77-412. 1961.
95. McFarland, J., and Meade, T. S. The genetic origin of tumors supported by their simultaneous and symmetrical occurrence in homologous twins. Am. J. Med. Sci. 184:66-80. 1932.
96. McKinnell, R. G., Deggins, B. A., and Labat, D. D. Transplantation of pluripotential nuclei from triploid frog tumors. Science 165:394-396. 1969.
97. Miller, E. C., and Miller, J. A. The presence and significance of bound aminoazo dyes in the livers of rats fed p-dimethylaminoazo-benzene. Cancer Res. 7:468-480. 1947.
98. Miller, J. A., and Miller, E. C. Chemical carcinogenesis: mechanisms and approaches to its control. J. Nat. Cancer Inst. 47: V-XIV. 1971.
99. Miller, R. W. Radiation-induced cancer. J. Nat. Cancer Inst. 49:1221-1227. 1972.
100. Mohr, U., Althoff, J., Kinzel, V., Süss, R., and Volm, M. Melanoma regression induced by "chalone": a new tumour inhibiting principle acting in vivo. Nature 220:138-139. 1968.
101. Monard, D., Solomon, F., Rentsch, M., and Gysin, R. Glia-induced morphological differentiation in neuroblastoma cells. Proc. Nat. Acad. Sci. U.S. 70:1894-1897. 1973.
102. Naegele, R. F., Granoff, A., and Darlington, R. W. The presence of the Lucké herpesvirus genome in induced tadpole tumors and its oncogenicity: Koch-Henle postulates fulfilled. Proc. Nat. Acad. Sci. U.S. 71:830-834. 1974.
103. Nichols, W. W., Levan, A., and Heneen, W. K. Studies on the role of viruses in somatic

mutation. Hereditas 57:365-368. 1967.

104. Noonan, K. D., Renger, H. C., Basilico, C., and Burger, M. M. Surface changes in temperature-sensitive simian virus 40-transformed cells. Proc. Nat. Acad. Sci. U.S. 70:347-349. 1973.

105. Nowell, P. C., and Hungerford, D. A. Chromosome studies in human leukemia. II. Chronic granulocytic leukemia. J. Nat. Cancer Inst. 27:1013-1035. 1961.

106. Old, L. J., and Boyse, E. A. Current enigmas in cancer research. The Harvey Lectures, Ser. 67(1971-72):273-315. 1973.

107. Oppenheimer, B. S., Oppenheimer, E. T., Stout, A. P. and Danishefsky, I. Malignant tumors resulting from embedding plastics in rodents. Science 118:305-306. 1953.

108. Ossowski, L., Unkeless, J. C., Tobia, A., Quigley, J. P., Rifkin, D. B., and Reich, E. An enzymatic function associated with transformation of fibroblasts by oncogenic viruses. II. Mammalian fibroblast cultures transformed by DNA and RNA tumor viruses. J. Exp. Med. 137:112-126. 1973.

109. Pierce, G. B., and Wallace, C. Differentiation of malignant to benign cells. Cancer Res. 31:127-134. 1971.

110. Pollack, R. E., Green, H., and Todaro, G. J. Growth control in cultured cells: selection of sublines with increased sensitivity to contact inhibition and decreased tumor-producing ability. Proc. Nat. Acad. Sci. U.S. 60:126-133. 1968.

111. Pott, P. Chirurgical Observations relative to the Cataract, the Polypus of the Nose, the Cancer of the Scrotum, the Different Kinds of Ruptures, and the Mortification of the Toes and Feet. 208 pp. Hawes, London, 1775.

112. Rabinowitz, Z., and Sachs, L. Reversion of properties in cells transformed by polyoma virus. Nature 220:1203-1206. 1968.

113. Rehn, L. Blasengeschwülste bei Fuchsin-Arbeitern. Arch. klin. Chirurgie 50:588-600. 1895.

114. Roberts, J. J., and Warwick, G. P. Covalent
     binding of 4-dimethylaminophenylazo-[3]H-
     benzene (butter yellow) metabolites with
     liver ribosomal RNA: the dissociation of
     the binding mechanism from the orotic acid
     incorporating system. Internat. J. Cancer
     1:573-578. 1966.
115. Rowley, J. D. A new consistent chromosomal
     abnormality in chronic myelogenous leukaemia
     identified by quinacrine fluorescence and
     Giemsa staining. Nature 243:290-293. 1973.
116. Rubin, H. Overgrowth stimulating factor
     released from Rous sarcoma cells. Science
     167:1271-1272. 1970.
117. Ruddle, F. H., Chen, T., Shows, T. B., and
     Silagi, S. Interstrain somatic cell hybrids
     in the mouse. Exp. Cell Res. 60:139-147.
     1970.
118. Rytömaa, T., and Kiviniemi, K. Control of
     granulocyte production. I. Chalone and
     antichalone, two specific humoral regulators.
     II. Mode of action of chalone and antichalone
     Cell Tissue Kinet. 1:329-340, 341-350. 1968.
119. Sacristán, M. D., and Melchers, G. The caryo-
     logical analysis of plants regenerated from
     tumorous and other callus cultures of
     tobacco. Molec. Gen. Genetics 105:317-333.
     1969.
120. Sambrook, J., Westphal, H., Srinivasan, P.
     R., and Dulbecco, R. The integrated state
     of viral DNA in SV40-transformed cells.
     Proc. Nat. Acad. Sci. U.S. 60:1288-1295.
     1968.
121. Scaletta, L. J., and Ephrussi, B. Hybridi-
     zation of normal and neoplastic cells in
     vitro. Nature 205:1169-1171. 1965.
122. Scher, C. D., Stathakos, D., and Antoniades,
     H. N. Dissociation of cell division
     stimulating capacity for Balb/c-3T3 from
     the insulin-like activity in human serum.
     Nature 247:279-281. 1974.
123. Schnebli, H. P., and Burger, M. M. Selective
     inhibition of growth of transformed cells
     by protease inhibitors. Proc. Nat. Acad.
     Sci. U.S. 69:3825-3827. 1972.
124. Setlow, R. B., Regan, J. D., German, J., and
     Carrier, W. L. Evidence that xeroderma

pigmentosum cells do not perform the first step in the repair of ultraviolet damage to their DNA. Proc. Nat. Acad. Sci. U.S. <u>64</u>: 1035-1041. 1969.

125. Shodell, M. Environmental stimuli in the progression of BHK/21 cells through the cell cycle. Proc. Nat. Acad. Sci. U.S. <u>69</u>:1455-1459. 1972.

126. Silagi, S. Hybridization of a malignant melanoma cell line with L cells <u>in vitro</u>. Cancer Res. <u>27</u>:1953-1960. 1967.

127. Silagi, S., and Bruce, S. A. Suppression of malignancy and differentiation in melanotic melanoma cells. Proc. Nat. Acad. Sci. U.S. <u>66</u>:72-78. 1970.

128. Smith, H. H. Plant genetic tumors. Progr. Exp. Tumor Res., vol. 15, Plant Tumor Res., p. 138-164. 1972.

129. Sorof, S., Young, E. M., McCue, M. M., and Fetterman, P. L. Zonal electrophoresis of the soluble proteins of liver and tumor in azo dye carcinogenesis. Cancer Res. <u>23</u>: 864-882. 1963.

130. Sorof, S., Young, E. M., Luongo, L., Kish, V. M. and Freed, J. J. Inhibition of cell multiplication <u>in vitro</u> by liver arginase. The Wistar Inst. Symp. Monogr. <u>7</u>:25-37. 1967.

131. Stephenson, J. R., Reynolds, R. K., and Aaronson, S. A. Characterization of morphologic revertants of murine and avian sarcoma virus-transformed cells. J. Virology <u>11</u>:218-222. 1973.

132. Stoker, M. Abortive transformation by polyoma virus. Nature <u>218</u>:234-238. 1968.

133. Swann, M. M. The control of cell division: A review. II. Special mechanisms. Cancer Res. <u>18</u>:1118-1160. November, 1958.

134. Symposium of the International Chalone Conference, 1st, Augusta, Mich., 1972. Chalones; concepts and current researches; proceedings. Proceedings editors: B. K. Forsher and J. C. Houck. 233 p. Bethesda, National Cancer Institute, c1973. (U.S. Nat. Cancer Inst. Monogr. no. 38)

135. Temin, H. M. Nature of the provirus of Rous sarcoma. U.S. Nat. Cancer Inst. Monogr. 17:557-570. 1964.

136. Temin, H. M. Control by factors in serum of multiplication of uninfected cells and cells infected and converted by avian sarcoma viruses. in Growth Regulating Substances for Animal Cells in Culture (V. Defendi & M. Stoker, eds.) p. 103-116. Wistar Inst. Press, Phila., 1967.

137. Temin, H. M. The protovirus hypothesis: speculations on the significance of RNA-directed DNA synthesis for normal development and for carcinogenesis. J. Nat. Cancer Inst. 46:III-VII. 1971.

138. Temin, H. M., and Mizutani, S. RNA-dependent DNA polymerase in virions of Rous sarcoma virus. Nature 226:1211-1213. 1970.

139. Todaro, G. J., and Huebner, R. J. The viral oncogene hypothesis: new evidence. Proc. Nat. Acad. Sci. U.S. 69:1009-1015. 1972.

140. Todaro, G. J., Lazar, G. K., and Green, H. The initiation of cell division in a contact-inhibited mammalian cell line. J. Cell. Comp. Physiol. 66:325-334. 1965.

141. Todaro, G. J., Green, H., and Swift, M. R. Susceptibility of human diploid fibroblast strains to transformation by SV40 virus. Science 153:1252-1254. 1966.

142. Toyoshima, K., and Vogt, P. K. Temperature sensitive mutants of an avian sarcoma virus. Virology 39:930-931. 1969.

143. U.S. National Program for the Conquest of Cancer. Report of the National Panel of Consultants on the Conquest of Cancer. Authorized by S. Res. 376 (agreed to by Senate April 27, 1970). Prepared for the Committee on Labor and Public Welfare, U.S. Senate. 150 p. U.S. Gov. Printing Office, Washington, D.C. 1970. (see page 100)

144. Unkeless, J. C., Tobia, A., Ossowski, L., Quigley, J. P., Rifkin, D. B., and Reich, E. An enzymatic function associated with transformation of fibroblasts by oncogenic viruses. I. Chick embryo fibroblast cultures transformed by avian RNA tumor viruses. J. Exp. Med. 137:85-111. 1973.

145. Varmus, H. E., Vogt, P. K., and Bishop, J. M. Integration of deoxyribonucleic acid specific for Rous sarcoma virus after infection of permissive and nonpermissive hosts. Proc. Nat. Acad. Sci. U.S. 70:3067-3071. 1973.

146. Verly, W. G., Deschamps, Y., Pushpathadam, J., and Desrosiers, M. The hepatic chalone. I. Assay method for the hormone and purification of the rabbit liver chalone. Canad. J. Biochem. 49:1376-1383. 1971.

147. Visfeldt, J. Transformation of sympathico-blastoma into ganglioneuroma. With a case report. Acta Pathol. Microbiol. Scand. 58:414-428. 1963.

148. Warburg, O. Versuche an überlebendem Carci-nomgewebe. Biochem. Z. 142:317-333. 1923.

149. Warburg, O. On respiratory impairment in cancer cells. Science 124:269-270. 1956.

150. Warren, L., Critchley, D., and Macpherson, I. Surface glycoproteins and glycolipids of chicken embryo cells transformed by a temperature-sensitive mutant of Rous sarcoma virus. Nature 235:275-277. 1972.

151. Warwick, G. P., and Roberts, J. J. Persistent binding of butter yellow metabolites to rat liver DNA. Nature 213:1206-1207. 1967.

152. Watkins, J. F., and Dulbecco, R. Production of SV40 virus in heterokaryons of transformed and susceptible cells. Proc. Nat. Acad. Sci. U.S. 58:1396-1403. 1967.

153. Weinhouse, S. On respiratory impairment in cancer cells. Science 124:267-269. 1956.

154. Weisburger, J. H., Yamamoto, R. S., Grantham, P. H., and Weisburger, E. K. Evidence that sulfate esters are key ultimate carcinogens from N-hydroxy-N-2-fluorenylacetamide. Proc. Am. Assoc. Cancer Res. 11:82, Abst. 325. 1970.

155. Whitfield, J. F., Rixon, R. H., MacManus, J. P. and Balk, S. D. Calcium, cyclic adenosine 3',5'-monophosphate, and the control of cell proliferation: a review. In Vitro 8:257-278. 1973.

156. Wickus, G. G., and Robbins, P. W. Plasma membrane proteins of normal and Rous sarcoma virus-transformed chick-embryo fibroblasts. Nature New Biol. 245:65-67. 1973.

162

157. Wiener, F., Klein, G., and Harris, H. The analysis of malignancy by cell fusion. III. Hybrids between diploid fibroblasts and other tumour cells. J. Cell Sci. 8:681-692. 1971.
158. Wood, H. N., and Braun, A. C. Studies on the regulation of certain essential biosynthetic systems in normal and crown-gall tumor cells. Proc. Nat. Acad. Sci. U.S. 47:1907-1913. 1961.
159. Wood, H. N., and Braun, A. C. Studies on the net uptake of solutes by normal and crown-gall tumor cells. Proc. Nat. Acad. Sci. U.S. 54:1532-1538. 1965.

ACKNOWLEDGMENTS

Acknowledgment is made to Columbia University Press for permission to reproduce in whole or in part the illustrations shown in Figures 1, 3, 5, 6, 12, and 14 of "The Cancer Problem; A Critical Analysis and Modern Synthesis," by Armin C. Braun, 1969; to Science for permission to reproduce Figure 1 of the article "Reversion in Hamster Cells Transformed by Rous Sarcoma Virus," by Ian Macpherson, Science Vol. 148, pp. 1731-1733, 25 June 1965, Copyright 1965 by the American Association for the Advancement of Science. The author should also like to express his gratitude to Drs. James S. Henderson, Ian Macpherson, and Roy E. Albert for making available original prints which have been reproduced in Figures 1, 7, and 10,B, respectively. The author also acknowledges support in the form of research grants from the National Cancer Institute, U.S. Public Health Service (PHS Grant No. CA-06346 and No. CA-13808) for studies on plant tumors the results of some of which are described herein.

INDEX

164

Horizons in Biochemistry and Biophysics

E. QUAGLIARIELLO, Editor-in-Chief, and
F. PALMIERI, Managing Editor (University of Bari)
T. P. SINGER, Consulting Editor (University of California, San Francisco, School of Medicine)

Contributors to Volumes 1 and 2

B. A. Ackrell	Pierre Desnuelle	P. J. F. Henderson	Paul Mueller
Daniel I. Arnon	Harvey F. Fisher	Ulrich Hopfer	John M. Palmer
Thomas B. Bradley, Jr.	S. Fleischer	Edna B. Kearney	J. Edwin Seegmiller
B. B. Buchanan	Irwin Fridovich	William C. Kenney	T. P. Singer
J. O. D. Coleman	M. Gutman	H. L. Kornberg	Donald A. Vessey
	H. W. Heldt	G. Meissner	David Zakim

The aim of *Horizons in Biochemistry and Biophysics* is to call the attention of students, teachers, and practicing scientists in the biological and physical sciences, including medicine, to

- major conceptual and methodological advances and important discoveries in biochemistry and biophysics
- the need for re-evaluating widely accepted theories
- the possibility of applying discoveries to knowledge in other fields.

In order to ensure the wide readership vital to the concept of the undertaking, the initial volumes of *Horizons* will be issued simultaneously in hardbound and in paperbound form. It is hoped that the relatively modest price for the paperbacks will allow individuals to enter *personal subscriptions*.

Volume 1, End 1974, about 350 pp., illus.;
   hardbound ISBN 0-201-02711
   paperbound ISBN 0-201-02721

Volume 2, Spring 1975, about 350 pp., illus.;
   hardbound ISBN 0-201-02712
   paperbound ISBN 0-201-02722

Continuation orders are invited.

Please place orders with your local bookseller or, in case of difficulty, with

ADDISON-WESLEY PUBLISHING COMPANY

Advanced Book Program	West End House	De Lairessestr 90	36 Prince Andrew Pl.	P.O. Box 363.
Reading, Massachusetts	11 Hills Place	Amsterdam 1007	Don Mills, Ontario	Crow's Nest N.S.W.2065
01867, U.S.A.	London W1R 2LR	The Netherlands	Canada	Australia